DI002907

Forty Days Off Facebook

A Pivotal Journey

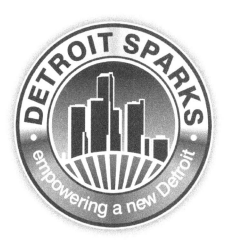

June 1st, 2018

WHY?

It has been 5 years since this book was published and almost 9 years since many of the events that I share in this journal occurred. Yet every time that I become aware that more students and people around the country will be reading this book, I do become self-conscious as this journal was never intended to be shared in this manner. Many people will judge the cover of this book and depending on their age and perspective may believe that the term "Facebook" is for old people. That may be the truth, however that is not what this book is about. I see my writings in this journal as a very unique lens and a snapshot in time within our civilization's history as social media, technology, and smartphones were beginning to collide with our society. Within this collision the symptoms of unresolved intergenerational patterns came to the surface along with the rising awareness of the importance of mental health.

Since this book has been published, many of the beliefs that I shared within these pages regarding addiction to social media and the impact that it would have on our society have come to fruition. Social media and Facebook had been utilized as a weapon by foreign countries to influence our elections as well as to enhance public discord. Over the past 10 years mental health issues such as anxiety, depression, and suicide have climbed significantly in direct correlation with the increase use and popularity of social apps and smartphones. Dozens of recent studies have been published highlighting the adverse effects on our sleep, our ability to maintain a healthy self-image, and our ability to maintain healthy relationships.

Before this book was originally published I had made several strong assertions in regards to the adverse effects that Facebook was going to have on our society from privacy issues to narcissism. My editor at the time strongly cautioned me that I was being too negative and that my assertions may turn people off. Even worse, they worried that I might become vulnerable to legal action from Facebook for making such claims.

Last month Mark Zuckerberg testified in front of government officials in Washington D.C. and in Europe in regards to the companies loss of personal data of nearly 87 million unknowing users, along with a host of other concerns. One individual in the European Parliament even went as far as to warn Zuckerberg that he could go down in history as the individual that destroyed western democracies. It's not fair to put it all on one person's shoulders, however the threat to individual privacy, and our data being maliciously used along with the effects that social technologies have on our society, has changed the course of history. We today are still trying to understand how to live harmoniously in this brave new world that has arrived so quickly and is here to stay.

This past month I was able to ask the former United States Surgeon General, Dr. David Satcher a question that I had burning within me. My question was: If he were still the United States Surgeon General today, would he consider putting a Surgeon General Warning on social media? After the audience gasped at the question, he answered, "I believed Zuckerberg would agree to some degree, obviously there are real dangers, and we need to say that. When not used appropriately, it can be very dangerous, and we are seeing that everyday. So, yeah, I would. When something is dangerous, we ought to say it."

At this time in our history we are awakening to the critical importance of mental health and how it connects to our physical body and world. The conversations are starting to change within media, within government, and within our homes. In the past few months it has been nearly impossible to turn on the television or plug into the web and not see a story of someone famous speaking about their own mental health struggles or hearing about another school that was put on lockdown because of threats of violence. The conversation and the reality is boiling to the surface. I do not personally believe this is a bad thing, I believe that we are going through a culture shift in which we will end up better off in the end. I believe that we are living in the era that will shift the tide and understanding of mental health as well as the body-mind connection. In 200 years from now, our ancestors are going to look back at these days and say that was when we became more aware of our reality. Similar to how we look back to the 1400's and find it hard to fathom that our ancestors believed the Earth was flat. The conversation is evolving and I, along with passionate allies, are honored to be a meaningful part of this change.

As you read the pages ahead I invite you to open your mind to how the world has changed over the past decade. I invite you to expand upon your curiosity without judgment of how each of us goes through life's trials and tribulations in our own unique way. My hope for you is that my experience from this time in my life plants a larger seed of awareness for how you choose to design your journey.

Sincerely,

Ryan G. Beale, M.A.

EDITORIAL LETTER
(Excerpts)
Forty Days Off Facebook, by Ryan G. Beale

Main Objective

The book's main objective is to document the author's own personal growth over a forty-day period during which he has stopped using Facebook. The intent is to document and work through his feelings at a period when significant anniversaries will fall—those of the finalization of his divorce from his first wife and the suicide of his brother Steve, both a year earlier.

The book is in the form of a journal, with almost-daily entries documenting events, thoughts, memories, dreams, goals, and regrets the author has during the forty-day period, and this is very successful at getting into the mind of the author and in telling the events of his life in the past few years.

However, it is less successful in its main purpose as indicated in the book's title: the reasons the author has decided to leave Facebook and what it is like to stay away from it. Given the title, the reader might expect daily reflections on what leaving Facebook has meant to the author (that is, what it's like to get along without it), and there are indeed some of those, but perhaps too few. The story might benefit more from further personal reflections of the author's own personal experiences on Facebook (and away from it) rather than lengthy examinations of why he thinks Facebook is bad.

The thesis tends instead toward sweeping pronouncements on the evils of Facebook and its founder, Mark Zuckerberg (see especially pp. xx-xx and xx–xx), and these detract from the overall story and lend an imbalance to it; almost nothing is said about the possible benefits or pleasures of Facebook or why people might choose to use it (instead, Facebook use is couched largely in terms of addiction, voyeurism, and stalking), and many readers (certainly those who themselves use Facebook, at least) will likely not relate to the overall thesis. Further, some of the assertions made about Facebook and Zuckerberg come across as potentially libelous (see p. xx–xx), or at very least unprofessional given that the author has started his own version of a social networking site, Chattertree. The book would, overall, benefit greatly from a more balanced presentation; and the negative assertions about Facebook and Zuckerberg need to be presented more as the author's own opinion and less as absolute fact, especially since no documentation is given to back them up (see comments on pp. xx–xx).

Tone and Style

The tone and writing style are informal, confessional, and self-reflective, and this approach is generally very effective given the personal nature of the subject and the journal form the book takes. However, as mentioned in the Main Objective section, above, where there are assertions made about the evils of Facebook and its founder Zuckerberg the narrative would benefit greatly if the writing had less of a preaching, condemning tone and more a tone of rational examination and exploration.

Other Comments

The causes behind the author's divorce and his brother's death are only touched upon, leaving a bit of a mystery for the reader. For instance, on page (xx) we read, "In the past year, I had lost a wife and a brother to uncontrolled addiction," and this might lead the reader to think that perhaps the ex-wife (and/or perhaps the author himself) and the brother may have had drug or drinking problems, but nowhere else in the book does it touch on what forms of addiction these significant life events entailed. On page (xx) we are told that the brother Steve has taken his life, but none of the circumstances of his suicide or what lead him to it are ever revealed. The narrative could benefit from a bit more fleshing out as regards these two very important events.

I hope these edits and comments are valuable in helping the manuscript achieve your publishing goals. Good luck in your revision, and I wish you all the best for this manuscript and future books!

—Brian, Editor

Forty Days Off Facebook
A Pivotal Journey

By
Ryan G. Beale

Disclaimer: The events depicted in this book are actual events written from the perspective of the author. The author and publisher have no direct affiliation with Facebook or the company other than being a user. Some of the names of people mentioned within this book have been changed to respect their privacy. The author has suggested that this book may not be suitable for children under the age of thirteen.

This book is available in quantity at special discounts for educators, organizations and retail distribution through the INGRAM Book Company www.ingramcontent.com

To learn more how your group or organization may benefit from this book please visit: www.40daysoff.com

Copyright © 2013 by Detroit Sparks, LLC
All rights reserved. No part of this book may be reproduced, scanned, or distributed in any printed or electronic form without permission.
First Edition: June 2013
Printed in the United States of America
ISBN: 978-0-98924-604-0

Cover Design by Ryan Beale

Dedication

This book is dedicated to the memory of my brother Steve, who always flattered me by telling me that I was a talented writer—right before he would make me write a speech for him.

(Written by the author and read as part of his brother's eulogy.)

My wish to you, Steve,

May your heart and mind forever be in peace
May your light shine and never cease
May your lessons become our education
May your dreams become our destination
May your family be left strong and left to thrive
May your friends and loved ones know that your spirit is with them and alive
May your heart reach the shores it was meant to reach
And may your life be a memory that we live to preach
I wish you all of the happiness that you were so desperately trying to find
And please look over us as our big brother in this very sad and challenging time

Love always and forever,
Smokey

Contents

Preface

If I were able to go back two years ago from today and share with myself the journey of what was to come, I could have never imagined the new beginning that was awaiting me. At the time I was somewhat confused and anxious. Looking back, I was most likely suffering from posttraumatic stress disorder. I had suffered a significant amount of tragic loss. The loss of my marriage, the loss of my home, the loss of my financial security, and my brother's tragic death were making me question reality. I had one goal, as those who supported me reminded me: be like an ark and keep above the waters until the storm clears.

Throughout my life many people have called me a dreamer. I have always found that dreaming is what gives our lives purpose. It is when we die that we stop dreaming, or at least we lose the ability to bring our ideals and dreams into the material world. I do have a few close friends who have been close to me long enough to realize that my dreams are not just mere dreams. They are early visions of my potential future life, filled with sweat, tears, prayers, and hope that with the right energy will start to manifest into something that leads to a happy future. If you dream big enough, you can be 100 percent certain to find some bashers along the way, but if you are lucky you will also find special people who will pat you on the back and continue to give you hope.

This project started off as a unique opportunity to keep a journal during a very anxious point in my life. I was hoping that it would work as a therapy to overcome what most would consider to be nothing short of "crazy" times.

I always dreamed of writing a book that could potentially open peoples' minds. I remember saying to myself when I started this experiment that depending on the outcome; I would consider making it into a book.

The reality is that what has transpired in my personal life since I started this self-therapy experiment is what I fear to be far more amazing than what I am capable of putting into words. This book is my best attempt to share the inner tribulations that led to the beginning of a whole new life chapter for me.

Meeting Facebook For The First Time

Click. Click. Click. Click. Click. Click.
Scroll
Scroll
Scroll
Click. Click. Click.
Scroll
Scroll
Click. Click. Click. Click. Click. Click. Click.

The whole family ran over to the whitish glow emanating from the laptop screen.

Click. Click. Click.
Scroll
Scroll
Click. Click. Click. Click. Click. Click. Click.

It was the late spring of 2006. My friend's little sister had just arrived back home from Indiana University for summer break. She was the first to introduce me to the world of Facebook.

Click. Click. Click.
Scroll
Scroll
Click. Click. Click. Click. Click. Click. Click.

I watched as her finger tapped the laptop's touchpad repeatedly. The response time was amazing. The next picture flew onto the screen instantaneously. The page didn't even reload between pictures. I was fascinated as pictures of attractive college girls partying in bikinis on spring break flew across the screen, one after another. The page load was less than two seconds. That was pretty impressive compared to my experience as one of the early adopters of Friendster. We eventually all started to outgrow Friendster and we soon began to ride the Myspace wave.

Myspace was starting to get a little too crowded at the time. I would regularly get spam from strangers, and the site's popularity was drawing tons of fake user profiles that were phishing for opportunity.

Seeing the speed of her finger and the response time of this new site, Facebook, left me speechless.

Click. Click. Click. Click. Click. Click.
Scroll
Scroll
Scroll
Click. Click. Click.
Scroll
Scroll
Click. Click. Click. Click. Click. Click. Click.

It reminded me of watching poor gray-haired ladies late at night in a casino in Vegas, the ones who look as if they are hypnotized by the slot machines. They will fight to the death if forced to leave that seat in front of the slot machine, even if the casino is on fire, their eyes and minds glued to the wheels of the slot machine turning and stopping, turning and stopping. It wouldn't matter to them if they had won a thousand coins or not. It was all about the next pull. It's this need that empowers the casinos to pay out 98 percent on most slot machines while still making huge profits.

Now it was the excitement of clicking the mouse or taping the touchpad rather than pulling a slot machine arm, not knowing what that next click might bring.

In psychology it has been well documented that if a reward stimulus is perceived as positive and is randomly given as opposed to regularly given, the likelihood for addiction is greatest.

We stood with family members and friends, waiting with excitement for the next picture to be exposed. It could be a snapshot of the neighbor's kid doing a keg stand. Maybe it was going to be someone passed out with a marker all over his or her face. Or just maybe the next picture would be their daughter wasted and sloshed on the floor. The excitement was contagious.

The volume of our voices grew and our attention was now focused exclusively on the laptop's monitor. Everybody was glued to it with the anticipation of what image would come next. What I saw was different, though; that this experience was game changing.

I knew that this was going to change the world of social networking and, more important, it was going to redefine how we connect and share as a society.

Facebook was not yet accessible without a college e-mail address, but as soon as they opened that gate I knew it was going to flood. What parent does not want to see his or her kid's college activities at their most unsupervised moments? What sibling who has been out of college for a couple of years does not want to connect with a little brother or sister? I would want to watch my little brother, if I had one, partying in college, and to have access to instant updates and thousands of pictures.

To me it was simple. The stimulus that could be achieved with this site was like nothing else available. To add to that, it was free.

My focus was going in another direction entirely. I had been working for the past several months on taking the power of the social network and trying to harness it into the soul of the family. We were going to name this courageous venture, Chattertree.

My goal was the complete opposite: I sensed an amazing opportunity to utilize this new technology to empower the psyche of the family. I mean, isn't that where the heart is? There is an energy that is created through the interaction of people in this new technology. It has the ability to awaken emotions through the instant connections and communications that are made.

The focus of family is where I was headed. I wanted to figure out the ingredients that would allow a family to connect, share, grow, and even heal together. Yes, I said it: "heal together." It was a challenge filled with passion and purpose. That was where I was headed and the power of the social network was what I was working with in order to harness that power.

I knew the wave that Facebook was going to create was on another level. It was satisfying, it was sexy, it was viral, and it was addictively smooth. It had the perfect ingredients for massive success.

I was aiming for modest success with evolving the family and the family system into a new level of inner harmony.

What does that even mean? It means that I believe that the family is the core of a peaceful and prosperous society. The family system is the collective function of the roles that family members take on. The family system works similar to how any organization works. In every part of our society you can observe systems and how they need to function properly when groups of people work together for a larger purpose.

If an organization such as the US Postal Service, the State Department, or an auto manufacturing factory had 25 percent of its workforce become dysfunctional, chaos would surely break out.

If 25 percent of post office employees in a major city didn't show up for work, you would have a complete snowball effect. People would become irate because of not receiving their important packages or letters on time; mail would be backed up; employees would become frustrated and irritable because they would be carrying the extra weight of those who didn't show up. And customers would end up mentally absorbing the employees' stress because of their lack of ability to fix the broken system fast enough.

The family system is also challenged and has a tendency to mentally break down at times. The breakdown is more likely to happen during times of high stress and tragedy.

We live in a society today in which, due to divorce alone, nearly 50 percent of all family systems are stressed and are not working as harmoniously they should. If you throw in statistics of families with members who are battling depression, posttraumatic stress, addiction, or confronting a cancer diagnosis, it becomes clear that the health of our family system is constantly being challenged.

Family is where the heart is. That being said, being connected and aware, and acknowledging the stresses within one's own family system, can be very difficult. It can be painful. It can be heartbreaking and even traumatic. Our ability to look within ourselves with pure honesty is a fair challenge. For the family group, honest reflection comes at a price. It can bring about the purest of emotions.

When you tap into the heart of a cohesive family system, all of the team members are unified in their quest for harmony. If they choose to work in sync with their values, customs, and expectations of each other, with a reasonable amount of flexibility for error, then harmony will be the end result of what the family system gives back to society.

It's a pretty deep conversation.

I personally believe that as a society we are living the generational effects that go back to the time of our biblical ancestors. We are carrying in our collective psyche the layers of their stressed—and at times broken—family systems.

Even Adam and Eve dealt with dysfunction in their family. Their son Cain killed his brother Abel. I mean, that's some real stress on the family system! There are documented sibling rivalries that have rippled down for thousands of years. I wonder what they did back then to heal.

Today the clashes of societies are between brothers, both sons of Abraham, who are caught up in a stressed family system that has created the sibling rivalry that we now see being played out in the Middle East.

The reality is that all of the issues that we do not do our best to resolve with harmony will be passed on to the next generation. If we don't work to find healthy solutions in order to purge ourselves of our inner unresolved anxieties, then we are doomed to pass that negative energy on to our families.

Young children don't understand where the anxiety is coming from, but they subconsciously learn coping skills at a very young age in order to manage the heavy stress on the family system.

Like an onion has layers upon layers upon layers, so too does a family. The family's layers are deep and sensitive. They are seen from an individual perspective and from a group perspective. They go back generations. Every time we can acknowledge, understand, and learn from the next layer, the closer we become to our core or soul.

These are some of the beliefs that fuel my position of why family is at the heart of society. These views come from my experience. Some of these issues I am pretty sure have been well documented and studied. Some of my viewpoints may be considered to be out of left field as regards modern family perspective.

Although I try to do research, to study and learn as much as possible, I acknowledge that I am not a doctor nor do I hold a professional title in the area of family system health.

I feel in my core that these beliefs that I hold come from a very pure and honest part of me. It feels at times that life has placed me in a position to observe, experience, and understand these latent lessons at a very deep and well-rounded level.

I have learned to respect that my life experiences so far are dwarfed in comparison to what some people must confront every day. Maybe, if I scream loud enough I can somehow help the conversation get out into the daylight. Who knows?

So that's Chattertree...and this is Facebook. One deals with the stimulus of opening up to family that you might not want to talk to, while the other can't wait to catch the neighbor fully exposed.

A couple months after seeing Facebook for the first time, I was sitting in a room with three investors listening to me pitch Chattertree and the power of the family network that we were creating. They were in their mid- to late fifties at the time; looking at me as I finished my well-prepared presentation they said, "We don't see how anybody over twenty-five is ever going to use this networking stuff! It all seems so young and childish."

I laughed; I knew what was coming.

The Facebook tidal wave was about to take them in—and their entire family with it.

I looked back at them and responded, "Mark my words, not only will you see twenty-five-year-olds using this, you will see people in their late thirties and forties, before you even knew what happened."

They didn't understand the power behind the network. That night they generously made us a low seven-figure offer to partner and I declined. I needed the partnership, I needed the cash, and I had the utmost respect for the guys that made the offer.

I was young and passionate. And I knew they did not have the patience to see this through. It would have been a "pump and dump." Full throttle until you run out of gas or you can buy the gas station.

I probably came off a little more confident than I intended to. I always recall that day and that meeting when my friend's grandparents request to be friends on Facebook.

My dealings with Facebook have lead to a complete love-hate relationship. I admire so many aspects of what has been accomplished because of Facebook over the years, but I am also affected by how it has stimulated a side of people that I feel is harmful to our society.

Four years later I was drowning in dysfunction, glued to the whitish glow of the screen and clicking away as if I was going to find something meaningful that would complete me. I knew better, but I still got sucked in.

Four Years Later

November 18, 2010

8:52 p.m.

Moments like these change your life forever and force you to decide how meaningful you want your journey to be. Are you going to be the victim, or you going to be the fighter? Are you going to design your future, or are you going to be a victim of the circumstances that surround you?

I am a fighter. I don't give up. My brother Steve was hard as hell on me and I know that nothing is just by chance. I need to be tough for what I am going to have to endure. I choose to fight so I can create and design my life the way that G-d wants it to be for me. I fight to find my larger purpose, so that I can leave behind something better than what was here before me.

As individuals, we all have something to offer this world that is so absolutely unique to our identities. Some will say that it is our divine purpose, to connect to this mission within ourselves. We must realize that there has never been a time in history, nor will there ever be a time in the future, that someone else will experience the same unique moments and opportunities that each of us can offer this world. Connecting to our unique footprint is the way we bring light into our lives and the world around us.

Get ready, because life is going to challenge your determination. It's going to challenge the strength of your mind. It's going to ask you if you are sure you want to fight for your dreams or if you want to choose a designated driver. When life throws a swing at me, I have to eat the punch sometimes, but I'm not going to let it knock me out.

I'm going to make a change.

Today, as insignificant as it may seem, I am making an attempt to do something that I have not been able to do in the past three years. I have noticed that I have an addiction and it is not the kind that I would have ever imagined. I have an addiction to Facebook and being plugged in to this thing now known as the social network. I say that I am addicted because I am no stranger to the pattern of addiction and what I call "the chase."— when you cannot sit still because you need more stimulation. The chase is what is obvious to observers on the outside when someone has a habit that is out of balance. The chase is what keeps us from connecting with ourselves and our deeper purpose.

We are all on a chase of one sort or another, and the chase is where we tend to find or lose our daily dose of purpose. It is what we are chasing that tends to be the problem. Some people are chasing money and riches, while others are chasing a good physique. Some chase spirituality, while others chase abundance in sex. Sometimes and unfortunately we tend to chase opposing goals at the same time. The problem is when we lose our awareness of what we are chasing and why we are chasing it. This is when we lose ourselves and we are basically driving the vehicle of our lives with a blindfold on.

These highs and lows are part of a pattern of addiction that hides itself in every little part of our society. Sometimes this pattern or cycle is hidden because the lows are not low enough to force us to change. That is when we get stuck, when the pattern becomes comfortable and even worse, socially acceptable. I lost my brother to the chase.

I now realize that I, like tens of millions of others, have become addicted to something very innocent, and that subtle chase today is Facebook. I have enjoyed the high of connecting with an old friend and the lows of not feeling the response I wanted from a picture that I just posted. They are highs and lows that affect my life, yet the severities have seemed so inconsequential that I have kept the pattern going. Why not? It's kind of addicting…

It took me a quiet moment and a memory of how comfortable patterns can hide themselves to realize that I may be caught a self-inflicted holding pattern. The memories of how these negative patterns have affected my life in the past is coming to mind. It is that pain that builds my courage to be willing to attempt to break the pattern. I was never aware in the past that I was stuck and that my personal growth was sitting—better yet, *sleeping*—and waiting on the sidelines for me to wake up.

One thing I have a challenge accepting is people who get stuck, become afraid of change, and give up on their dreams. I am not going to allow my circumstances to become my destiny. I am going to undertake a project. The only way that I am going to be able to test how much something is affecting me is to remove it from my behavior and keep a working log of my thoughts.

I have decided to embark on a project to break the seemingly innocent yet dangerous cycle that I believe may be delaying and holding back my life potential. If I am correct, I will realize new potential when I am done and a new door in my life will begin to open.

My project is to conserve the energy that I exhaust on observing other people's lives through Facebook. I am going to do this at a very challenging time and when I know anxiety and stress will kick in during the anniversaries of some of the most significant and symbolic days of my life thus far.

These are times that will bring my tragedies and trauma to the forefront of my mind. I believe that Facebook has had the potential to keep me lost in an unhealthy behavioral cycle. I also know from experience that it has not bared much fruit toward the quality of my life other than spamming out postings for business.

I'm going to keep a living journal of this process over the next forty days. If my hypothesis is correct and I stick to it, I will have removed an addiction and allowed true personal growth to resume.

November 19th, 2010
3:41 p.m.

You're probably asking, why choose to take forty days off Facebook. I'm asking myself the same question. What is the purpose? My reasoning is that forty days has always been a historic time frame between an old chapter ending and a new one beginning. For me, these next forty days will bring the anniversaries of some of the most pivotal, and hardest, times in my life.

Here is some of the fascinating historic and religious symbolism that comes with the number 40: See http://en.wikipedia.org/wiki/40_(number).

Judaism

- Rain fell for "forty days and forty nights" during the Great Flood.
- Spies explored the land of Israel for forty days (Numbers 13).
- The Hebrew people lived in the Sinai Desert for forty years.
- Moses' life is divided into three forty-year segments, separated by his fleeing from Egypt and his return to lead his people out.
- Several Jewish leaders and kings are said to have ruled for forty years. (Examples: Eli, Saul, David, and Solomon.)
- Goliath challenged the Israelites twice a day for forty days before David defeated him.
- Moses spent three consecutive periods of forty days and forty nights on Mount Sinai.

- A *mikvah* consists of forty *se'ah* (approximately two hundred gallons) of water.
- Forty lashes were one of the punishments said to be meted out by the Sanhedrin (though in actual practice only thirty-nine lashes were administered).
- One of the prerequisites for a man to study the Kabbalah is that he be forty years old.

Christianity

- Before the temptation of Christ, Jesus fasted forty days and forty nights in the Judean Desert.
- Forty days was the period from the resurrection of Jesus to his ascension.
- In modern Christian practice, Lent consists of the forty days preceding Easter. In much of Western Christianity, Sundays are excluded from the count; in Eastern Christianity, Sundays are included.
- In the Old Testament, it rained for forty days and forty nights in the Great Flood in which all land-dwelling living beings perished except those on Noah's ark.

Islam

- Muhammad was forty years old when he first received the revelation delivered by the archangel Gabriel.
- Masih as-Dajjal roams around the Earth in forty days, a period of time that has also been expressed as forty months, forty years, and so on.
- The Quran states that a person is only fully grown when they reach the age of forty.

- Musa Moses traveled forty years in the desert, and spent forty days on Mount Sinai, where he received the Ten Commandments.
- Prophet Ibrahim spent forty days in a fire and lived because Allah made the fire like flowers.
- In the fortieth verse (*aya*t) of the second chapter of the Quran (Al-Baqarah), Allah changes the topic.
- Forty was the number of days that prophet Ilyas Elijah spent in the wilderness before the angel appeared to him with Allah's message on Mount Horeb.
- Forty was the number of days that prophet Isa Jesus was tempted in the desert by Satan.
- Muhammad prayed and fasted in a cave for forty days. He then had forty followers to spread the religion of Islam.
- Prophets Dauud and Suleiman each ruled for forty years.
- Regarding the flood that Noah encountered, it is said that for forty days water continued to pour from the heavens and to stream out over the earth.
- There is also a hadith from Muhammad that the prayers of a person who gossips would not be accepted for forty days and nights. (Al-Kafi 6:400)
- Imam Ali has narrated from Muhammad that one who memorizes and preserves forty hadith relating to their religious needs shall be raised by Allah as a learned scholar on the Day of Resurrection.
- It is said that a person's intellect attains maturity in forty years, each according to his own capacity.
- It is believed that one who assists a blind man for forty steps becomes worthy of entering heaven.
- Imam Baghir has said, "The prayers of someone who drinks wine are not accepted for forty days."

- Believers have also been encouraged to devote themselves to Allah for forty days to see the springs of wisdom break forth from their hearts and flow from their tongues.

Yazidism

- In the Yazidi faith, The Chermera Temple (meaning "forty men" in the Yazidi dialect) is so old that no one remembers how it came to have that name but it is believed to derive from the burial of forty men on the mountaintop site.

Russian Folklore

- Some Russians believe that ghosts of the dead linger at the site of their death for forty days.

Hinduism

- In Hinduism, some popular religious prayers consist of forty *shlokas* or *dohas* (couplets, stanzas), the most common being the Hanuman Chalisa (*chaalis* is the Hindi term for forty).
- Some of the popular fasting periods consist of forty days and are called periods of *Mandl kal*. (*Kal* means a period of forty days.) For example, the devotees of Swami Ayyappa, the a Hindu god very popular in Kerala, India, strictly observe forty days of fasting, with their offerings following on the forty-first day or a convenient day after the minimum forty-day fast. The offering is called *Kanikka*.

Forty Is Also...

- An Arabic proverb: "To understand a people, you must live among them for forty days."
- The caliber of the bullet in a number of firearms cartridges, most notably the .40 Smith & Wesson. The 10mm Auto, although designated as metric, uses the same caliber and often the same bullets.
- The saying "Life begins at forty."
- The expression "forty winks," meaning a short sleep.
- The number of years of marriage designated as the ruby wedding anniversary.
- The dialing code for international phone calls to Romania.
- The number in the designation of
  - Interstate 40, a highway that runs from California to North Carolina.
  - US Route 40, the 2,285-mile (3,677-km) highway that runs from Baltimore, Maryland, to Park City, Utah, a portion of which follows the National Road.
  - European route E40, which runs from Calais, France, to Ridder, Kazakhstan.
  - The A40 and M40, important highways in the United Kingdom. The A40 is a trunk road in England and Wales, connecting London to Fishguard. The M40 motorway is the second motorway in the British transport network to connect London to Birmingham.
- A song ("#40") by the Dave Matthews Band.
- A song ("40") by the band U2.

- A song ("40'") by the band Franz Ferdinand.
- The number of ounces in a bottle of malt liquor referenced in the song "40 oz. to Freedom" by the band Sublime.
- A visual term for rural Ireland, "forty shades of green." Johnny Cash popularized it with a 1961 song of the name. The band Crush 40 (composed of Johnny Gioeli and Jun Senoue) from the *Sonic the Hedgehog* video game franchise.
- The stage name of Canadian hip-hop producer Noah Shebib, "40."
- The number of thieves in "Ali Baba and the Forty Thieves" and "Ali Shar and Zumurrud" from the *Thousand and One Nights*; both the numbers 40 and 1001 are more likely to mean "many" than to indicate a specific number.
- The customary number of hours in a regular workweek in many Western countries.
- The number of positions on a number of radio countdown programs, most notably *American Top 40*, *American Country Countdown*, and *Rick Dees' Weekly Top 40*.
- The budget ($40) on *The Early Show* segment "Chef on a Shoestring."
- The number of weeks for an average term of pregnancy, counting from a woman's last menstrual period.

A Final Fun Fact

Forty is the only number that, when spelled out, has all its' letters in alphabetical order.

Moving Forward

Over the next forty days I will experience the anniversaries of several life-altering events that Facebook has somehow influenced or for which it has served as some sort of veiled coping mechanism. It has become a source of anxiety, addiction, sadness, joy, voyeurism, stress, and exhibitionism.

I want to experience what my life will be like over the next forty days when I commit to unplugging from the social network. I will reflect upon my past, my dreams, and lessons learned. This challenge will, I believe, lead to a journey—one that I need to walk through, one that will allow me to leap into my future and will start to heal wounds from the past. The first thing I need to do is to deal with the alligator closest to the boat, that which is preventing me from true self-sufficiency. Today that closest threat is the one that Facebook inherently exploits.

I'm going to document my raw thoughts and emotions in what I would simply like to call my *personal pure mental graffiti*.

Master Reset
November 19, 2010
5:26 p.m.

My status update: Taking forty days off Facebook to connect. If you want to reach me just give me a call or e-mail me
—All the best.

Day 1
November 20, 2010

8:45 a.m.

I woke up this morning knowing my routine has to be changed.

On a normal day, I would wake up in my one bedroom River North apartment, curiously check the weather by peering over the western Chicago skyline, and would make my way to the bathroom. Somehow I would find myself walking over to the computer, half dressed while I started checking out the news. I would click on the latest Facebook newsfeed and then refresh it to see what everyone had to say that morning. I always started my day reaching out to see what was going on around me. Even on a good day I often forgot to reach *within* and start my morning with what I wanted to accomplish that day. I soon realized that I had forgotten to take full advantage of that day and, most important, the start of it.

I am embarrassed to say it, as silly as it sounds, but last night I started to feel some effects of physiological withdrawal from signing out of Facebook. The first occasion was while I was driving over the La Salle Bridge, which sits upon the Chicago River. I saw the most amazing view of the nearly full moon over the colorful lit up Wrigley Building, showing off its awe-inspiring green halo. It was nothing short of breathtaking. I caught myself in the act: instead of inhaling that moment the way it was meant to be, as a gift to me, my initial knee-jerk reaction was "That would be a great picture to post to my Facebook page." I laughed at myself knowing that I was aware of my first challenge in this journey.

At that moment I took a deep breath and looked at the moon over the green, lit-up Wrigley Building. It was absolutely amazing, a scene right out of one of the Batman movies, the kind that the directors would have spent hundreds of hours on in order to portray the perfect Gotham City night. I took another breath and enjoyed my serene moment.

This morning I'm going to work to turn off the constant outflow of energy that is constantly demanded of us, at least for a moment. I'm going to say a prayer for my family, my friends, and myself.

4:15 p.m.

I caught myself in tears watching *Avatar* on HBO right now. I remember when I first saw this movie in the theater. It was literally right after my brother died. The movie started off with the soldier's brother dying, and the brother had to come to take his place; there was no one else for the job. At the time I had felt that this was an eerie parallel hitting me, but I was still in shock then. Now, watching almost a year later, I realize that I have been spending a lot of energy trying to avoid confronting the pain and the grief.

I know that I have Facebook at the top of my mind, especially during this project; however, it's already becoming more clearly aware that I have been using it as a coping mechanism. It has been a way for me to connect and see what everyone else is up to rather than looking deeper within. It has distracted me from allowing the grief and the stress to take their natural course.

It was a good distraction for some time, but I know there are repercussions that arise from keeping your mind distracted and from not connecting to your soul. Addictions do not have to be in the form of a substance, such as a pill or a bottle, to damage your mind. We use many habits in life to withdraw from ourselves like a drug. Things are starting to feel just a little more real, as I am only beginning to remove the inhibitors.

Day 2
November 21, 2010

9:35 a.m.

If you asked my friends what my bizarre hidden talent might be, there would be little question that they would answer that it is remembering dates. I do my best to walk through life with my eyes wide open, and for whatever reason, anniversaries and birthdays have always tended to stick in my mind. Throughout this journey, this will happen often. This is why these forty days are so impactful to me; the anniversaries start today.

Last night I was walking to dinner for my friend Julie's birthday, which happens to be today. Julie was my first girlfriend after I filed for divorce, which was May 14, 2009. We met a few months later on August 13. Julie had come out on my boat as a guest of my friend Fred's girlfriend. I wanted to take three months after filing for divorce before I was willing to go on a date with a girl. Thankfully my ex and I did not have any children, but I still felt I'd give it three months before I would open myself to the dating scene once again.

I saw that Jason Mraz was playing at the Charter One Pavilion on the near south side of the city. It was on the evening of my three-month anniversary from filing. I was thinking it would be a great opportunity to take the boat out for an August summer evening to see that concert. I did not have a date going into it, but thanks to Fred's suggestion, Julie was adventurous and available, that night could not have been more perfect.

The concert was awesome, and we fell hard in the

moment. Julie and I ended up dating for the next three months. I was still trying to get my divorce finalized throughout this time. It was a tough balance. Julie and I enjoyed each other and respected each other, but it ended when I realized, "What the hell am I doing, jumping so fast into another relationship before I am healed from the last one?" Add a couple crazy episodes, a little insecurity, the threat of a never-ending divorce process, and a sexy little lady to that equation and you are guaranteed a recipe for disaster.

What was I thinking? There is no way that after nearly two years of complete chaos in my marriage was I ready to open myself up and allow myself to be fully vulnerable again. Julie and I were not meant to be partners, which we learned by default.

I was weak at the time and I will admit she was a strong and powerful little lady. She had her own ideals and I had mine on how things should be in a healthy relationship. The truth was, we were both just trying to learn from our past experiences and mistakes. It was too soon for me. Julie had my number, she was able to scratch at my core, it was too soon, and I was too sensitive to chaos.

It was October 17, right before my friends' wedding, that I said enough and literally put her on a train from Detroit, where we were visiting, back to Chicago. Yeah, kind of harsh, but she told me that she had a lot more respect for me after that. I think she saw me getting so beat up that she was surprised I still had some fight left in me.

The relationship was a risk I took and learned from, and once I realized it was toxic for both of us I cut it off. This was a lesson that I have had to remind myself about. Somehow I completely blinded myself in my past marriage. I'm still trying to figure it out. I did not see the red flags, or at times I intentionally ignored them. Either way, a lesson must be learned to move forward properly. I am thankful to say that Julie and I remain great friends since that night when I put her on a one-way ticket back to Chicago.

Being that I am an individual who often allows numbers to connect to my memory and emotion, I found it fascinating that Julie was born on the same day, same year, and in the same hospital as my ex-wife. When we went to dinner at Julie's house for the first time to meet her parents I drove as we went twenty-five miles north of Chicago; we took the exit I was accustomed to, but instead of turning left toward where my prior in-laws lived, we turned right and went to Julie's parents' house.

It was beyond bizarre, and a part of me feels that it was not by chance, either. When we first started dating, I thought maybe something got mixed up (upstairs) and I got the wrong one at first. So today is Julie's birthday, my ex's birthday, and my wonderful Old English sheepdog Jack's birthday. To say I've given my heart to November 21 would be an understatement.

Thankfully, today I will call my friend and wish her a happy birthday. As for my ex-wife, I would call her, but not this year. Tonight I will look forward to driving back to Michigan later this week to see my parents for Thanksgiving, and maybe I'll cook up a steak dinner to give to Jack for his birthday.

Looking on the bright side of things, I don't have to worry about posting cold birthday messages nor be a voyeur on anybody's updates. Although we don't talk anymore, my ex and I still for some reason remain Facebook friends.

11:45 p.m.

Just got home from dinner with friends for Julie's birthday. Of course, she and my ex-wife both chose the same restaurant in which to celebrate their birthdays this evening. I politely left after dinner to avoid adding any potential negative energy to the night; there already was a full moon. No need to stay around and soak up the awkwardness of the evening. Good night.

Day 3

I'm feeling slightly like some balance is starting to shift as I avoid using the computer and my phone to see what everybody else is doing or what I'm missing out on.

I took a great photo today that was very meaningful to me. The thought of sharing it on Facebook ran through my mind. If it is meaningful to me, why not share it, right? Just the fact that the picture was relevant to me and maybe a few people that would get the inside joke does not mean it needs to be shared. I'm catching myself.

I am realizing more and more that we are being constantly trained and reminded to keep up with the Joneses. Everything we want to show off or exploit and blast out to our personal public comes from a sense of our need for relevance from the outside. Unfortunately, there is a very large audience of people that want to see, evaluate, and judge, and—if we are lucky—they will comment on our public notices to give us proof of relevance.

I've been able to live through several life cycles in the short time I've been using Facebook. I've used it as a man who was "in a relationship," as one who was "married," and back again to "single." I've also used it as a utility to push out business dealings, to gain some attention to my ventures.

Each cycle in the past couple of years has had Facebook's fingerprints all over it. Looking back, every Facebook activity I took part in had a slight dose of anxiety and a small amount of nervous energy that was part of it. It is not something that would normally raise the alarm levels, but I realize the subtle anxiety within myself and I see it in everyone around me.

There is an addictive behavioral undertone that is propelling this significant movement online. There is always a subtle constant feeling and internal void from the continuous need to check in and see if others have responded. This is usually followed by a slight low if no one has responded or shown any love. Other times there is a huge high to some degree to see that people appreciate what you have to offer or show. It tends to be a subtle energy drain and a time filler to see what other people are doing.

I tend to wonder if people are being genuine in their pictures and messaging and how much are they staging for the sake of public consumption. There is no doubt that it is human nature to mask our genuine emotion in order to exploit what we are creating for public consumption.

Either way, speaking for myself, I feel more and more that it is something that is pulling me away from my center. Facebook is pulling me away from enjoying a healthier balance, and that is why I feel it is fair to equate it to an addiction. The user constantly wants more, without a sense of full satisfaction.

Day 4
November 23, 2010

11:59 p.m.

I'm writing to keep my consistency and discipline sound. I need to be able to reflect for myself, and hopefully others may benefit from my experience during this forty-day journal-writing period. Today was the first day I really did not have any anxiety. Usually there is a slight build of anxiety when someone's name comes up and I have the ability with my phone to view his or her profile with my friends, show pictures, see how we know a person, and cast judgments.

Today Facebook came up twice in conversation where I was asked to pull somebody's profile up. They looked at me like I was crazy when I told them I was taking a vacation from Facebook. My friends asked if I was really that addicted and if it was that big of an issue for me. When I explained that I believed it was something that is adding unnecessary noise at this point in my life, I actually got great responses. It was empowering for me. I could tell that everybody related to that fact that we are all just a little caught up in maintaining our profiles.

It is amazing to have to the ability to connect to an old friend and/or stalk someone in a matter of seconds. I am enjoying how much more rewarding it is to have real conversations about life with people I care about. Today I was able to do just that. I'm beginning to build connections just from talking with others, discussing things and laughing at ourselves. It felt like my soul was more alive.

Day 5

Tonight, the eve of Thanksgiving, is known to be the biggest bar night of the year; it is a pretty big deal in the suburbs of Detroit. With the mass exodus from the Detroit area over the past decade or so, it's anticipated as a night of reunions. It is the night when all of the people who left Michigan come together from all over the country to hang, be seen, and do everything they can to avoid getting pulled over while driving home after a long night of drinking.

I have been doing my best to keep a positive mind-set. Nights like this have become hard for me because I can feel the heaviness in people's eyes gazing at me when I come back home. This was by far my brother Steve's favorite night of the year next to Halloween. He was a rock star in this town, and this is the first year of not experiencing him throwing the party and sharing Thanksgiving with us.

I keep recalling last year and where I was for Thanksgiving and how bizarre the circumstances were at the time. My parents went to Florida because my grandmother was not doing well. For years I had wished I could have a quiet meal with my brother Steve without twenty people and 20 other distractions around. I could never get him to sit still unless he was sleeping.

Last year my Thanksgiving dinner was at his home with just Steve, his girlfriend, and myself. It was the most enjoyable and relaxing meal I have ever had with my brother. Unfortunately, we spent a good amount of the evening talking about my ex-wife and how he had felt that her family was taking advantage of the divorce process. He was bothered how they had involved and burdened my family in this ordeal.

Steve was concerned how my ex was not willing to sit down to close this painful chapter. There was concerns shared that inaccurate claims were potentially being made on court documents. It was prolonging what was already a very sad and drawn-out situation.

I remember that we had just found out that my ex had crashed my car a few weeks prior. It had come to my attention that the accident had sent several people to the hospital and had been hidden from me. It only became revealed once I received a call from the insurance company asking if we had changed our address. I had tracked down where my car was that week. It was ready for pick up after six weeks of being repaired. I had to race to claim my car from the repair shop before it could become another point of contention.

There were fifteen thousand dollars in repairs to a car that I bought for just over twelve thousand dollars. It was another reminder of how toxic the marriage was. I was going to be named on a lawsuit that I had no part of. On paper we were still an entity. I had begged and pleaded for my car back for months just for that reason. I had written letters to the family begging for us to just be able to move on. This was the reality that I had been living with since I got married. No matter where I was, there was some tragedy brewing that I was not aware of, yet I had full responsibility and liability to clean up the broken pieces.

That night, last year, I remember my brother being frustrated and bothered. I think Steve was trying to protect me from the emotional anguish of the divorce. He always would push me to make sure I was doing everything I could to move the process along. It was adding unnecessary stress to all of us.

The conversation soon shifted to my plans for the weekend. This was the conversation that I try to remember most. We lost ourselves in outrageous laughter about the fact that I had a somewhat blind date after dinner. It was going to be a first date with my big Old English Sheepdog puppy, Jack. We all could visualize how Jack's aggressive attention hoarding was going to—for sure—kill my game; my dog was so damn hyper and needy. We laughed about him nonstop. When I was newly single, Jack soon became known as instant lady repellent. My brother's girlfriend made it a point to let me know that if I wanted anything to do with this girl I needed to do something to chill this dog out. Jack is great and only full of love, but she was right.

Throughout this conversation, filled with chuckles and outright laughter, the idea of Benadryl crept into the conversation. I thought they were joking, but they were so serious. I knew they were right. If I wanted to have a good first date, I needed to be proactive, and I was convinced to do something about it. I left Steve's house as fast as I could to find a store, any store that would have what I needed to give my dog to make him chill out.

I found some Benadryl tablets and I tacked on some string

cheese to the local 7-11 bill. This is probably, in theory, one of the more cruel things I had ever done to my dog Jack, but it was with good intentions. I just needed to give him something that would make him a little sleepy so I could enjoy my date night.

Bottom line, it didn't work at all. Jack was more hyper than he had ever been in his life. He was running all over the room, barking for attention, and he kept leaning on my date, begging to be rubbed with his red rocket at attention. It made for good conversation throughout the date, although I never shared the fact that I mildly tried to drug my dog so I could enjoy my date's company.

That was the last time I saw my brother alive.

Day 6
November 25, 2010
10:59 p.m.

I just got done watching the roast of David Hasselhoff on Comedy Central. It was a gift of ninety minutes filled with feel-good laughs. I appreciated his ability to get roasted while maintaining his integrity. He ended with the exact quote that embraced my thoughts of what today meant, saying in his slightly cheesy Hasselhoff tone, "Remember, sometimes life will give you a wake up call. It's about how fast you get up, not how hard you fall."

That quote hits home. It feels much like what my day-to-day and my life have become. Today was Thanksgiving. It was full of good friends, highs, lows, growth, sadness, family, and hope.

I woke up early on my friend's couch after going out for the big bar night before Thanksgiving. After about four hours of sleep I woke up and took a stroll outside. It was a nice coincidence to realize as soon as I opened the front door that my old Chicago roommate, Alex, lived across the street. I guess this is not such a unique phenomenon in good old downtown Birmingham, Michigan.

In both houses, people were getting ready to spend the day with their families. They had their days planned, running from one family member's house to another. I had realized that I did not want to leave. Even as they were getting ready to go, I tried to delay the inevitable. I knew that once I left, I had to live my new Thanksgiving reality alone.

In the past year, I had lost a wife and a brother, both to circumstances that were beyond my control. I had lost my wife's family as well, which I knew and loved as family for a good part of my adult life. All but a very small handful of her friends had pretty much turned a cold shoulder to me once I filed for divorce. The hardest part of the breakup was friends taking sides. Nobody wanted to be caught in the middle. By the reaction I received from some of our close friends after our marriage came to a halt, I was pretty confident that I was made out to be the villain. My brother's death just added to the depth of these stories.

The distance that old friends had shown did not surprise me, nobody other than myself had taken on any of the responsibility during the marriage, why should the divorce have been any different. The distance of the friends that had taken sides crushed me most after loosing my brother. I needed the added support. My support circle had been cut in half, if not more.

When I needed the support of my family, their world had been rocked by the loss of my brother as well and they now needed their own support. It has just been one vicious cycle after another. Thank G-d we did not have any children.

After spending so much of my energy working to save my marriage, it had continued to eat at me how people I genuinely loved and cared for, now had different eyes for me. They were like family to me. I was feeling more isolated than I had ever been in my life.

I had lost my brother permanently.

My ex-wife hopefully will live a healthier and more meaningful life, but my marriage died and that devastated me. The grief was deep. Losing my wife and my dream of a family was and continues to be a grieving process for me.

I know that one day I will find love and build a family again with G-d's help, but losing a big brother so tragically is a fact that I still have to remind myself, daily, is my new reality. I try to understand and learn from the pain with the hope that there is something powerful that can come out of this tragedy.

This morning as I left my friends and they all got into their vehicles to see their families, I became overwhelmed with extreme sadness. To think that this year my Thanksgiving dinner was just going to be my mom, my dad, and myself. Last year it was just my brother Steve and his girlfriend. These two dinners by far are the quietest Thanksgiving dinners I have ever experienced.

My brother Sam and his family are in North Carolina but to ask that they travel with two kids and a third on the way is a little too much at this time. I knew this year was going to be extremely difficult to reach the level of fun, liveliness, and silliness that we used to all once enjoy. As my friends all drove off, I walked with a soldier like step toward my car door, opened it up, and sat down; a little bit of my heart swallowed itself.

I got into my car and drove directly to Einstein Bagels. There, at my favorite quick breakfast spot, I grabbed my regular: egg whites on a toasted whole-grain bagel and a large vanilla hazelnut coffee. I started drinking the coffee, contemplating how to make the most out of this day, which was going to end with a Thanksgiving dinner for three. The idea of the previous year's dinner being the last time I saw my brother alive kept coming in and out of mind as everybody around me was elated and enjoying this special day with their families.

I chose to embrace my fear and anxiety and allowed it to push me through the day as a curious journey. I got into my car and started driving east toward the cemetery. It took me about a half hour to get there. It was not until I saw the exit was coming up that my heart and my tears started working in sync. I pulled into the cemetery, and as I drove toward my brother's plot, I slowly passed a family paying the grave of their loved one a Thanksgiving visit. There were five of them standing there, with arms around each others backs, kids and all. My gut told me they were visiting their father's resting place.

I drove along the narrow road, and as I passed we all made eye contact as if the day was being played in slow motion. We shared in that moment a look of understanding that though pieces of our hearts were gone for eternity, we could still give thanks for the pieces we had been left with.

I pulled up to the secluded area where my family had several plots. My great-grandparents, my grandfather, my uncle, and now my brother rest in this quiet place just a couple hundred feet from the road. I walked by slowly and paid my respects to the souls who had brought me here. After walking by all of their plots, I just wanted to be close to my big brother, so I sat directly behind his headstone.

He had been so hard on me growing up, but no matter how tough he was I had still always wanted to be by his side. He wanted me to be tough, and he always taught me to stand up for myself and to fight back if people tried to put me in a corner.

I use to be so upset with him and how he could be so hurtful to me. I realize now more than ever, that he had his own internal struggles. As little brother, I took a significant amount of the anger that he was holding onto. At this point in my life I could thank him because without his tough and tormenting love I would never have been able to get through these difficult times. This was the second time I had visited his grave since the funeral. The previous time was right after his headstone was put up. Seeing our shared last name on my brother's headstone had then put my system into shock; I was a sobbing mess. This time I felt more at peace.

My brother was always on the move. The guy must have had red ants in his pants 24/7. Throughout our shared lives, I had never been able to sit next to my brother and share my inner thoughts with him without getting a fierce tongue-lashing. I could never just sit and enjoy a peaceful silence with him. It breaks my heart that we had challenges enjoying a silence together while he was alive, but I have chosen to find and embrace the positive influences and lessons he gave me through his tough love.

When visiting a gravesite, it is a Jewish tradition to leave a pebble or a rock on the headstone to show your respect to the dead and that you have visited. I once heard that it was symbolic of the destruction of the Old Temple. The last time I had been at the cemetery I could not find any stones or pebbles, so I went into my car and grabbed the only thing that made sense. It was a piece of clay that I had from a prior trip to Israel, from the city of David, that I kept it in my car for good luck.

The piece of pottery clay was said to be nearly two thousand years old. I stomped on the piece of clay and it broke into five pieces. It was exactly one piece for each of my family member's gravesites. I was happy and moved to see that all the pieces still sat on top of the five headstones where I had placed them several months back.

I left the cemetery, passing by the family again. I headed west back toward my parents' house; it was getting close to dinnertime. I was starting to feel connected; connected to purpose, connected to life, connected to death, connected to reality, and humbled. I felt slightly somber.

As I was driving towards my parents, I felt like Steve had given me a sign. My passion project, Chattertree, was given a great mention online for Thanksgiving. I have spent the last four years of my life working on ideas and tools that would help families become closer. Selfishly, I wanted it to help my family the most.

Chattertree had started from an idea of creating a heartfelt gift for my father. I was looking to do something special to surprise him for his birthday. I was thinking about creating a blog that could work as a living tribute to him. I was going to post pictures of some his personal milestones.

After my father had beaten non-invasive bladder cancer at the age of fifty-one, he spent his energy teaching his three sons about going after their dreams. He did this through leading by example.

Throughout my father's life he had always loved bodybuilding and always dreamed of competing in it. He recommitted to this childhood dream after his wake-up call, and started training three to four hours a day. He had befriended world-class bodybuilders who pushed him farther than he had ever gone before.

He had seen that the All-Natural Iron Man competition was coming up in a few months. To reduce his chances of backing out, he told everyone he knew that he was going to be competing. He committed additionally by buying tickets for nearly thirty of his closest family friends.

My father worked out like a machine. Standing only five feet six inches, he was solid as a rock. He weighed only 150 pounds or so, with a twenty-eight inch waist, but he could bench press 350 pounds.

The day of the competition had arrived and my father was looking great. He was in the best shape he'd ever been. As we walked up to the theater to register, the other competitors started getting out of their cars.

One by one, these lifelong body builders started coming up and crowding the registration line. I think that these other guys may have not seen the print on the event title, which clearly stated: "All-Natural".

These guys looked like that had eaten boulders for

breakfast. My dad looked at me and I looked back into his eyes. The silence spoke volumes. The lesson that he was teaching had been conveyed.

No matter what happens in life, we have to push ourselves and fight for our dreams. There is always going to be someone who will make you question your place in this world. There is always going to be someone who is stronger, smarter, and wealthier.

It is not about how we compete with others; it is about how we challenge ourselves and how we define what it is to be strong, wise, and wealthy.

I had met recently with a rabbi who was discussing this topic. The rabbi asked, "How do we define someone who is strong, someone who is rich, someone who is wise, and someone who is honorable?"

The thoughts that came up were fascinating. In society we tend to dictate these categories based on creating a correlation to others. The bottom line is that we tend to chase strength, wisdom, and wealth in order to achieve honor. This chase is something that is damaging to our state of mind.

When it came to strength at the local gym, my father was out-benching the trainers. Once we arrived at the theater and in a room full of only guys that eat boulders for breakfast, he was not considered to be the one who stood out.

The same goes for wealth and wisdom. There is always going to be a room full of more that will leave you feeling like less. In regard to honor, if you picked up and moved to a place where you did not know anyone, how would they know that you are honorable?

The perspective on this topic was simple, yet rich with depth. It has been said that one who is strong is one who has conquered his or her inclinations; that one who is wise is one who chooses to always learn from the lessons of other people and life experiences; and one who is rich is one who is happy with his or her lot in life. And finally, one who is honorable is one who honors all others.

The day my father got on that stage in his competition Speedo and with his artificial tan, the humility of these lessons was understood.

I wanted so badly to put the picture of him on stage in his full flex on the blog that I was thinking about making for him. That picture meant so much to him and to me, but for reasons other people would never understand.

That is where the ideas started evolving. It needed to be private. I did not want others to judge or laugh at something that meant so much to both of us. I thought, *What if his blog had a password? Who would we share the password with? What if we wanted to have private conversations—would we include the people that we had given the password to?* The questions kept evolving, and so did the solutions.

I have been investing my soul into Chattertree while I slowly and painfully witnessed my own idea of family die and transform.

As I looked at the Google analytics from my iPhone, the site was getting tens of thousands of hits. To see this brought on a great natural high. It was all because of Kim Commando, a radio host who gave Chattertree a three-page write-up as the "tip of the day" for families on Thanksgiving to use. What an awesome feeling that was!

Kim has no idea how she and her timing positively uplifted me.

At times, life tends to throw us signs that we are in the right place at the right time and that, no matter what cloud is overhead, the sun will still peek through. It was very refreshing to have a stranger from across the country give tribute to a project that has come from the depth of my being and tears filled with experience. This little notice and boost to Chattertree came at such a perfect time and was truly a gift while I was feeling most vulnerable.

I am thankful that when it storms in life and the storm takes away our home and fogs our faith there is always a new day on the horizon. Sometimes, if we are looking hard enough, we will even see a rainbow. We just have to walk through the rain, and when it storms, we have to convince ourselves to find a way to dance.

Day 7

"Black Friday." I just thought, what would I be doing right now if I were using Facebook? I probably would be getting spammed with hundreds of notices on my friends' feeds about attending the blowout sales. I'm excited that the economy is feeling a sense of vibrancy again, but these "shop all night" advertisements and people by the thousands waiting outside in the freezing cold for the doors to open make me laugh at how we play along like junkies.

Today I woke up with a voice mail from a local magazine writer who wants to do a story on Chattertree. I am fairly nervous yet confidently enthusiastic about the opportunity. This will be my first real interview. I have no clue what they are going to ask and what questions may unknowingly provoke my heart to start pouring out. I am so close to Chattertree, and ever since my brother's passing, helping families connect and be healthier has become a life mission; it is a great vessel through which I can promote a positive message.

I have been staying at our family cottage. It is a small quaint summer home on Cass Lake that my parents bought nearly twenty-five years ago. I have spent a significant part of my life there. It's where I can be alone at times and reflect while enjoying the water. The winters are more somber as the lake freezes and life seems to slow down quite a bit. The cottage is where I stayed most of the time when I came home from Michigan State University, and later Chicago, for the weekends. Being just 7.2 miles from my parent's house in West Bloomfield, it's close enough to stay close yet far enough to still maintain my independence and freedom.

As I left our family cottage today, I looked into the mirror and smiled. I was starting for the first time to see my true self without the veil of shock, sorrow, and the past. I smiled and knew now that today I was living in the moment. I walked outside and our first snow was lightly falling; a new season was emerging.

Day 8
November 27, 2010
10:59 a.m.

Got tagged in a photo. Just got the e-mail notification from Facebook—so annoying, and I can't check to see what it is. Another gentle reminder of why I hate Facebook at times.

Day 9: – Back to Chicago
November 28, 2010

Day 10
November 29, 2010

1:45 p.m.

The past two days have given me an insight into where I need to position myself for future success. I am not talking about just financial success, however, but success also in emotional matters, relationships, and in finding confidence and focusing on goals. Financial success, I believe, will be the byproduct of all these aspects working in harmony based on my DNA and my natural energy being in sync.

It started by getting a touch of humility this past Saturday evening when I was still in Michigan. I also found it quite interesting that the day seemed to be surrounded by conversations in regard to the power that can be gained through an insult. Earlier in the week I picked up a book that had once belonged to my grandfather, *The Gateway to Happiness*. I did not feel like reading the whole book, so I just opened it to a random page, which started off by asserting that if we can change our perception of an insult from anger or frustration and think of it instead as a blessing, then we can use that humility to push us in the right direction. Then we can look at an insult and say thank you.

Earlier on Saturday, a woman who I am a friends with had opened a different book and showed me a sentence that she had underlined—it was this same message. I smiled, as I saw this as a nice coincidence that has been resting, not far down in my subconscious.

That evening I walked into my friend's house and his

twenty-three-year-old girlfriend proceeded to tell me that I had come up in conversation between her and her friends. They had been gossiping, and even went to the extent of calling *me* a whore. My first reaction was, ouch!

My ego was slightly bruised and my oversensitive side started feeling over-compassionate that I may have hurt someone's feelings. My father frequently tells me that we are always judging peoples actions yet we should look deeper at people's intentions. Intentions are where the heart lies; actions are often faulted by human error.

Over the past year I have started to date again after my very painful and difficult short marriage and an even more painful divorce. I wanted to see what people were about, and I needed to practice letting my guard down as I was healing. For some reason, I became entranced with twenty-three-year-old women from the same area as my good friend Danny's girlfriend. While they were all mutual friends on Facebook, I wasn't sure if this was actually the case in real life.

I think I was naturally drawn to this group of young ladies because they were attractive and fun, and we shared new perspectives and an entrepreneurial spirit; and that was exciting. Twenty-three-year-olds are often searching for identity in the world. They are vigorously trying to find their balance in life among their careers, their passions, and their reality. I guess it's fair to say that in that respect, I too was in a newfound search for some of those same things. As my friends put it, I was acting as sensitive as a twenty-three-year-old.

I actually found it refreshing that women in this age group

did not require me to be as emotionally available as women closer to my age did. There was a sense of freedom and a free spirit that I needed to heal from my divorce and the trauma of losing my brother. It was working. It started opening my heart again and, at times, my heart overflowed.

I was always concerned that my contact with one of the women from the past year would come to hurt my chances of getting to know someone that I might see a future with. I wrestled with this. I wanted to date and meet as many people as I could before I decided to team up with my next life partner. I'm thirty-one and divorced, with a zest for life, a heart of gold, and a natural fathering instinct, and if you asked my parents they would tell you I am quite handsome as well. I don't want to make the same mistakes twice. Putting myself out there was the only way I knew how to make forward progress in the field of opening myself up to future true love.

Well, on this past Saturday night my fear came true. Although I was not hooking up with any of these women at the time, nor had I in the past, the fact that I was trying to pursue friendships and possibly more was enough to fill up the conversation at the dinner table. E-mails in which I had attempted to open up during low points had come back to bite me.

The thoughts and feelings that I had shared via e-mail reflected some of my insecurities at the time, but this group of twenty-three-year-old women interpreted them as my attempt to "play" everybody. Hence the "whore" comment that came up in the same sentence as my name. When I first heard that this is how I was perceived, I was hurt and felt insulted; but I soon realized that I needed to learn a lesson from this.

The friend who gave me the heads up felt terrible that I was sad and taken back by the information. She kept saying that she was sorry, but I stopped her, saying, "No, thank you." Remembering the lessons earlier that day from the book The *Gateway to Happiness*, I knew that I needed to hear it.

I made a choice at that moment to grow up. There is a time for young fun and there is a time to learn and live. It was now time for the latter. I never wanted to hurt someone, nor be the joke of a dinner party but, like every other lesson, I will take the insult as a gift, awakening me to a more fulfilling tomorrow.

3:10 p.m.

I just slipped. It was for the first time and it was really quick. I logged in to Facebook to become a stalker. I wanted to try and see pictures of a girl I had met over the weekend. I started getting the voyeur bug, which made me feel like an outsider to the gossip circle, and then I cut myself off to get back to me.

4:31 p.m.

Second worst f***ing call of my life! A college fraternity brother just called and told me that his big brother has killed himself. He asked me what he should do. I stayed calm and was honest as every image of the call I got about my own brother came to mind. I told him his body and mind are going to go into complete shock and he needs to remember that this is the first part of the grieving process, that he needs to take care of his mind and start doing mental push-ups to fight off the anxiety.

He asked if I would be around later; I said of course. I hung up and then yelled, "F**k!! That's all I could remember when I got the call about my brother. I was a zombie, packing to head back home after the holidays, and all I could do was yell "F**k!" I lost him. I could not save my brother. Those feelings for my friend are breaking my heart right now.

I just hope that some of the lessons and coping tools I've learned can help him and others through challenging times. I told him that he has a choice, to allow the experience to break him or to allow it to define him. He is strong, with a good heart. I have confidence that this tragedy will define his character and somehow will bring him to a place he could have never gotten to without this life lesson.

Day 11

11:30 a.m.

I started my day with a sense of sadness for what my friend and his family must be going through. It definitely brought out a lot of feelings of sadness, anger, and even rage. Thank G-d I got back into martial arts. It has been a great outlct for helping to maintain balance in my life. Last night I went to my Haganah class and let out some of my unanticipated aggression.[1] It helped me sleep through the night and allowed my mind to rest and reset. I'm lucky I have defined a mission in my life.

That mission is to be happy and to help others. Chattertree has been my coping mechanism for negative energy and life frustrations, and it has allowed me to create something positive that has the potential to impact millions of people and families. Today when I woke up I remembered my friend and then I remembered my mission.

As usual, I ate a great breakfast, one so large it could easily feed two people. I love a good breakfast; it prepares me to enjoy the day. It gives me a chance to relax, reflect, and catch up on either a book that I am reading or the latest news.

---

[1] Haganah is primarily a mix of Israeli martial arts—called Krav Maga and Hisardut—and Israeli military systems. All are blended together in a unique way so that only the strongest most tactically sound approaches from each system are used.

Today I had to prep for my first phone interview for Chattertree. The site is more than a business for me; it is personal; it has become a life mission. There is great power behind social technology; my mission continues to be to harness the greater good within society. I believe that resides within the individual, but can be harnessed from within the family unit.

Social networking is our modern revolution. It amazes me to think about the historical impact of this newfound technology on society. How we use these new advances has so much potential for the greater good or for the exact opposite. In almost all circumstances, it is spread out across both.

For example, rocket propulsion is an amazing advancement for modern-day society that can be used to take people to the moon or to explore the universe; or it can be used to create a ballistic missile to create destruction and bring fear to people's minds thousands of miles away.

Understanding nuclear energy has allowed us to have the ability to give power to a whole city, or it can be used to wipe out an entire city in seconds. Although these are drastic examples, this is how I view the current trend of social networking. It can be used to connect us and bring us closer or it can be used to create a voyeuristic, addictive society that will ultimately make us feel more alienated from each other.

I fear that this is what Facebook is doing to our modern society. There is a false sense of closeness because genuine connections are far and few between. Our information is being shared, and that can alienate us from genuine intimacy with others and a sense of self-understanding. People feel that they know each other before they have even met. The younger generation and now the older generations are beginning to use social networking as an alternative to having real-life connections. Outsiders are pulling our attention away from real issues and we are becoming quietly addicted, like members of a blind cult.

I personally do not know one person who is on Facebook who, when he gets an e-mail saying he was tagged in a random photo, does not automatically have a sense of ants in the pants. I would bet that the average person's blood pressure, if measured, it will increase as soon as he gets that e-mail. Feelings of curiosity, worry, and human insecurity can tap so delicately into the psyche.

Mark Zuckerberg was brilliant in his execution. In my opinion, he was able to precisely get into the psyche of the user. In time, I believe people will forget and/or become numb to the negative draws that got them hooked in the first place. I believe people will also find it ironic that their personal lives are being shared in ways they never anticipated. That's where people will most likely learn to understand the cost of something that is said to be "free".

When I would sign off from Facebook, Friendster and even Myspace back in the day, I always felt slightly drained. It was as if I was left with an unfulfilled void in my heart. I would tend to get a little itchy and come back for a little more. I was aimlessly hoping to fill the whole. It is subtle, but it was there.

I tried to relive this message in my phone interview today, but the feelings of sadness toward my friend's recent loss and my own tended to overshadow the conversation. The interviewer said she had done a little research and found out that my brother had committed suicide. She asked if she could talk about it with me and write about it, acknowledging that it was a sensitive subject. My response was that as long as my experience can benefit others then I feel a sense of obligation to discuss the heaviness of the topic.

6:05pm

I feel that in every experience you must learn a lesson and make it a priority to take that lesson and make it a part of your life. I believe that if you take the lesson and use it to do good, to help others and the world within which we live, you will reap the rewards in this lifetime. Religion often preaches that you will have your place in the world to come, but I have faith *today*. Although I am struggling through the closing chapter of difficult times I have faith that my good deeds and good intentions will come back around and will ultimately help shape my life for a more positive and rewarding future.

I have also made a pact with myself that I will do everything possible to make this a reality. My heart and my intentions are only good and often have been misinterpreted in ways that have challenged me at every stage of my life, so I fight forward.

I was talking to a woman that I am friends with about relationships and about allowing ourselves to take a breath in between relationships to learn a few lessons.

People are so often afraid to be alone that they are willing to sacrifice a lifetime of fulfilling happiness by settling for the quick fix. It is our addictive nature and anxiety that drives us to make those quick-comfort decisions to accept less than we deserve out of fear.

We talked, and I genuinely wanted her to understand the lessons that can come from a failed relationship. I started to fear that she would not respect my thoughts on the issue because I was divorced. I have friends that rebut out of anger and frustration—they say, "What do you know? *You* got divorced." In my heart that sense of failure will always have a scar, but I never will doubt my commitment to making my relationship work. I was not going to allow my past to dictate my future.

I was aware of my moments in which I had to battle frustration, heartache and dishonesty. I ultimately made a decision for two people to be happy in the long run. I had to give it up when I knew there was no more fight left in me and the man upstairs would never approve of me being so miserable and useless.

I told my friend from the bottom of my heart that I know a lot about "love." I know about anger, I know about hate, rage, sickness, and compassion, and I know about love. I also went on to explain that nearly thirteen years of my life was filled with falling in love, being in love, fighting for love, and then trying to fight my way out of love.

I could speak of it because I was conscious of it. I knew that in sharing love, someone was willing to open her heart and share it with me. I wanted to truly respect her by learning from her and embrace her in every way that I knew how. I did this so I could grow as an individual and we could grow closer together. That was always my hope and, at times, maybe my fantasy.

My high school girlfriend was my best friend for several years prior. She was confident, and always wanted to help people. She had this beautiful, vulnerable, best friend, don't-get-in-my-way vibe that I was drawn to. We were awesome together, sidekicks running the party. When college got in the way and started pulling us apart, it was the most painful experience I had ever had. It was my first love. She made me realize that I needed to grow up. I do not know if she ever knew this, but she helped me find my smile, and because of her I learned to laugh more.

In college I dated a girl for three and a half years. I am thankful for the gift of confidence that she gave me. She was a beautiful, sexy blonde, five foot three, a second-degree black belt who rode a Harley. She also was a 4.0 student, and wanted to grow up to be the real Lara Croft. I kid you not, she could have done it if she had stayed on that path. She pushed me into a life of martial arts. She also pushed me to get rid of my crotch rocket at the age of nineteen and trade it in for a more mature Honda Shadow 1100. In my junior year at Michigan State, when I was at a crossroads, about to step away from a group of guys I had put together to restart a failed fraternity, she looked at me and said, "You need to run this." I wanted to walk away and focus on our relationship and just enjoy the rest of college, but she pushed me to be a leader. The fraternity members nominated and voted for me to be the re-founding president. That led to one of the best experiences of my life. Loving relationships had changed my life, and since then it has continuously enabled me to grow.

Day 12

Just took off from Midway Airport, and I am flying above the clouds on my way to Fort Lauderdale to spend the next five days with my brother's old best friend, Rick, who has been like a brother to me. It's also going to be family time in south Florida. The driving force behind this trip is the fact that my cousin is getting married. With family spread all over the country, it has been a challenge to get everybody together. Although dysfunctional at times, we're still family.

I am looking most forward to spending quality time with my grandmother. The wisdom and life lessons of the elders are some of the most treasured moments in my life. If they can still share a genuine smile, then they probably also have a valuable lesson you can learn. The genuine smile is usually the best indicator. It shows that they are at peace with themselves, have accepted the challenges of life, and have embraced the reality of death.

Grumpy old folks, on the other hand, will tell you stories that are usually filled with hardship, tragedy, and dissatisfaction with the past. The thing I often find most interesting is that these two diametrically opposed types of individuals can often be found as life partners, married and sharing the same highs and lows. Yet one type has chosen to take their G-d-given talent to look through different eyes and learn lessons, while those of the other type tend to see themselves as victims.

My grandmother is my role model in this lesson. My

grandfather was a sergeant in World War II, stationed in Alaska and later had several unsuccessful businesses. They lost their son tragically when he was thirty-eight and they shared in almost every experience aside from the war. The various hardships they experienced could easily have led to my grandfather's hardened views. My grandmother was always sweet and welcoming, but she was scared to step in the wrong direction and set my grandfather off.

He loved us and cared deeply for all of us, but he could be a mean, angry son of a b**ch if you crossed him or set him off. When my grandfather passed away just over a decade ago, it was like my grandmother's cocoon was popped wide open and the liveliest butterfly came flying out. She was the life of the party, at the center of every dance circle at any celebration. People would talk for weeks prior to an event about how they could not wait to see grandma Carmen get up and shake her bum. She started singing at her neighborhood events and writing poetry in the local newsletters. Her spirit lit up every room she set foot in.

She and I share such honest conversations about life they would probably make an old dog's ears perk up. She has taught me to live my dreams, to love even when it is hard, to sing even when the acoustics are not perfect, and to dance my ass off. She has reminded me that I can't wait a lifetime for things to work out to start to live; I must learn to dance in the rain. Over the past couple years her body has not been able to keep up with her spirit, and I know in my heart that she's getting ready to let her body go so her spirit can dance. I think the only reason she has been holding on is because she wants my family to heal enough before she leaves us. She is at peace with herself, and that is why I try to learn from her. I want to take advantage of every lesson and every moment that I can bask in her spirit. These precious moments I can selfishly take hold of, allowing them to enhance the rest of my life.

5:45 p.m.

I had to pull myself away from the TV to make a note from earlier in the day. As I just pulled myself away and "unplugged" I walked out onto the balcony with my journal and overlooked the Atlantic Ocean from the thirty-ninth floor in Hallandale Beach, Florida, at my friend Rick's. I can hear the ocean hitting the sand from here; the sky is a navy blue just before dusk yet I can still see the horizon. Water has a healing power like no other and it has always been a significant part of my life. As I write this, memories of writing next to water in journals since I was a teenager are flashing through my mind. I am recalling in my subconscious that my dream has always been to be able to write and live by the water. This has been a vision of mine for a fulfilling retirement. I have always wanted to write something meaningful that could help empower others. Who knows? Maybe there is a chance that this could be one of those books that I always dreamed of writing. I still don't know what will come out of me and what I may learn by the end of this forty-day journey.

Getting back to why I got away from the TV to write a note: I realize that my relationships in the last week and a half are beginning to take on more depth. My ability to connect with a stranger and the energy I put out to that person is becoming much more welcoming and meaningful. In the past twenty-four hours I talked with two separate people for about two and a half hours each. We talked about life, culture, and goals, religion and relationships, parenting, marriage, divorce—*real* talk, the kind we all yearn for, yet we tend to be either too afraid to open up or are too anxious to sit still and listen.

On the way down here, I sat on the plane and talked with a seventy-five-year-old Italian lady about the lessons she learned. Oh boy, did she have lot to talk about! It was a wonderful coincidence, because my last entry, about taking advantage of learning from the elders, was almost an exact reflection of this conversation that was now naturally taking place. That is why I think it is important to take note that real connections that nurture my core are evolving. I am feeling more connected and more settled. I believe it is because I am more aware of myself and I am making a conscious effort to stop looking outside myself so often for fulfillment.

Day 13

December 2, 2010

6:50 p.m.

Sitting in the same spot I was yesterday as I made my last entry, I ask myself why am I not living closer to the warmth and the water. What is wrong with me? Right now it is 20 degrees and snowing in Chicago—too cold to do much of anything. In the Midwest, wintertime always tends to get tough on the mind. The days are shorter, the trees shed their leaves, people lose their summer glow, and the fact that we sit in our cars for ten minutes shaking and making funny shivering noises makes me laugh. Just the lack of vitamin D from the sun is enough to put anyone in a slight funk.

It makes sense that so many religions have a holiday centered on the idea of adding lights this time of year. The holidays of lights would seem to have become the rebranded theme of all major religions. With dark nights starting so early, it is important to try to lift the spirits. I just find it ironic how the holidays are branded to be so joyous, filled with gifts and splurging on food. There's a lot of pressure when your heart is heavy and you are still grieving the loss of a loved one. My heart goes out to the families who are struggling with loss or feeling pressure to get their children gifts they cannot afford. I guess I can see how these things can create a high-pressure opportunity for individuals to self-reflect. If they do not entirely break someone who is struggling, they might actually help push him or her in a meaningful direction. This year, for me the holidays are a reminder of what matters.

Days 14–15: Discovery
December 3–4, 2010

Day 16: Understanding Trouble

December 5, 2010

3:30 p.m.

Over the past couple of days I have spent a significant amount of time reflecting on my childhood. My past has come back to challenge me. I am starting to think that this was the purpose of why I randomly picked the page in that book *The Gateway to Happiness* that had talked about allowing insults to positively form you and how to learn to accept and appreciate them. It was almost as if I was being prepped for what was to come.

I met this great woman when I was back in Detroit; she is in a phase of rediscovery herself. She just got out of a long, challenging relationship and has an amazing outlook on life that I am drawn to. She too was grieving in her heart. She had a close girl friend that was brutally murdered earlier in the year by a guy that her friend was hanging out with. We are relating emotionally at a deep level of understanding to the loss of long relationships and the tragic loss of a loved one.

I see her beautifully optimistic outlook on life and I see her yearning to grow from her pain. We have naturally been drawn to each other because of it.

The first thing she did after we met was ask me to be Facebook friends. She was temporarily denied. It is a breath of fresh air to have to get to know someone before you can just pry right into every aspect of her public profile. It has given us a chance to talk on the phone about the things that matter most without having visuals of each other's past experiences at our fingertips.

I am enjoying this old-fashioned approach, one that is becoming less and less common these days. Over the past week she had mentioned my name to a couple of friends and coworkers of hers. They both know me from afar or from my childhood, and their first response to her was, "He's trouble!"

Thankfully she is confident and strong enough to think independently. She also has a sense of adventure and curiosity, which may help my chances.

Growing up, I had two older brothers and an array of influences. The neighborhood I grew up in in the changing suburb of Southfield, Michigan, was a little more street savvy than my later neighborhood of West Bloomfield, which had a high density of isolated upper-classers.

I got myself into a good amount of trouble before I was even a teenager. I was the kid that caused more gossip than harm most of the time, but my actions sure did create conversation for the masses when we moved to West Bloomfield.

If someone else was doing something wrong and I was there, I usually ended up taking the full blame just because it was expected of me. It was already understood that I was the kid coming from a middle-class neighborhood with older brothers, and conversations about my personal experiences seemed to be enjoyable dinner table fodder for those with little to talk about.

People all walk in their own shoes, yet for some reason everybody seems to understand where you are coming from. It amazes me how closed off we are as a society and that we often allow singular events to define people that we only know from afar. I have lived through this scrutiny in my life, starting at a very young age. Unfortunately, I created unneeded attention to myself on several occasions. My actions as a youth created obstacles for me that I still have to confront now in my thirties.

When I was nine years old, my brothers—sixteen and fourteen at the time, started gambling in the house with their friends. Being the youngest of the siblings, all I wanted to do was to hang out with the boys, no matter what that entailed. I would sit on the corner all day selling lemonade to make a few bucks with the hope that they would see me as a relevant card player. Those hard-earned dollars would only last me a few hands before my long days' work was equal to zero.

Feeling helpless, I would hide in my closet and cry with frustration, not understanding the full range of my emotions. I was nine years old at the time, for heaven's sake. I had just lost the money that I hustled all day for and, even more painfully, I had lost the opportunity to prove relevance.

All I wanted to do is to be part of the gang. The idea of winning some money added a level of excitement that I chased. I had learned math faster than most of my friends and I knew how to shuffle better than most casino dealers by the time I was ten. Selling lemonade had turned into selling baseball cards and running sports card trade shows by the age of twelve. The chase unfortunately became part of my personality.

I was looking for stimulation, with a goal of getting my next rush, being with the big boys, and making a strong statement of relevance. Looking back now with more maturity, I know with 100 percent certainty that I was on the chase.

My purpose was to feel like I was a player in the game who had a potential upside. When I would lose, I would be devastated. I would cry alone, hiding it from my parents, and over the years that hidden shame would transfer into anger that always got me into trouble. I always ended up at the wrong place at the wrong time. It took me nearly eighteen years to break the cycle of that chase. I had to realize that when you are chasing the never-lasting moment, you lose site of your true self and what a real connection with yourself and others means.

Working all day, only to lose later what I had earned, taught me about the pattern most addictive gamblers get stuck in: the feeling that no matter how broke you are or how dim things look right now, you'll still have enough breath to make a comeback tomorrow.

This high and low is a pattern of addiction that hides itself in every little part of our society. Sometimes this pattern or cycle is very hard to find because the lows are just not low enough to force us to change. That's when we get stuck, when the pattern becomes comfortable and, even worse, socially acceptable.

Throughout my adult life I have always attempted to look at every significant event and ask myself if there is a lesson I need to learn. How did this event make me feel, and what can I take away—either positive or negative—

from this experience?

I am asking myself now why does it bother me today that people still define me on the basis of situations from my childhood? I know that I have had to endure some painful lessons, but I have faith that these lessons were meant to build my character as an adult and would define my unique life. We are not all meant to be alike.

I'm definitely sensitive about the gossip that encircles me because it could affect me getting to know someone who might mean something to me today. In my heart I know that people can gain from the lessons of my experiences. However, if people choose to judge me based on a bad moment or my actions as a troubled youth crying out for attention, then my message of lessons learned will not only *not* reach them but will have the consequential effect of making me doubt myself. In life, if we doubt ourselves because of other people's judgments, then we become slaves to social acceptance and abandon our dreams. Pursuing our dreams, or even just *some* of our dreams, is what gives us a larger sense of purpose.

You will not find too many people on their deathbeds saying that the one regret they have in their fleeting life is that they followed their dreams too often. Rather, you will find the opposite. You will find that some of the top regrets of people at the end of their lives is that they focused too much on what other people thought of them, worried about social acceptability, and focused too much on making money. I would rather fight for a greater, more meaningful purpose than become a slave to the chase.

I am working on channeling that criticism that was aired

today into positive energy to help me push further than I would have been able to do without having heard these negative judgments.

My brother Steve taught me, through harsh lessons at times, how to fight even though it feels like the world's odds are stacked against you. He also taught me how to gamble, so I have been spending my time and energy away from the tables and using that energy to gamble on myself, my ideas, and my potential to help someone else live with a little more perspective and hopefully slightly less heartache because of something I had endured.

I am hopeful that because my intentions and my actions are coming more in line with where my heart is, that G-d will bless me with success in this venture in my life.

Day 17: Back to Chicago
December 6, 2010

Day 18

I just got a healthy dose of anxiety. Thankfully I'm using it to push myself to write what I am feeling and thinking at my core. A friend and I were discussing Chattertree and talked about the importance of privacy, how we want to make the site child safe and make sure it is a site that the whole family can connect to and feel comfortable at. During the conversation my friend mentioned that he'd heard Mark Zuckerberg had been on *60 Minutes* and asked if I had seen it. I had not, although I usually watch the show, so being intrigued, I Googled it. Business aside, when I watch Mark Zuckerberg speak, my blood pressure must jump 50 percent or more. What he has accomplished is amazing. There is no doubt he is brilliant. But what he lacks is genuine life experience and he has created a monster that is taking over our society in such an unhealthy way. It eats at me. Social networking is creating ambivalence on a scale that is destroying our real bonds and relationships with each other. I am not confident at this point in his life that Zuckerberg fully understands what value genuine emotional connections have on the human spirit.

As I see it, Facebook is teaching us how to judge each other in an instant, sidetracking us from the true journey of what makes us human and numbing our spiritual side. Our privacy is going to be sold to the highest bidder and we are going to be tracked in ways we never could have imagined ten years ago. The fact that Zuckerberg is on *60 Minutes*, asking people to trust their family to his creation is something that makes me quite sick. Yet, I know that most people will jump in with blinders on, along for the ride because they already have their toe in the Facebook waters and social addiction feeds the ego better than anything.

There is always an outcry on the part of its users when Facebook privacy guidelines change (as they often do), much like a child will cry when he instinctively knows something is not right. The users then become pacified and continue along. I pray that this is not where society ends up. I am fearful that we are all just going to become a database of our social lives—a cold number with snapshots and blurbs lacking genuine substance. We cannot be defined as the data-fed voyeurs and exhibitionists that we are becoming. Zuckerberg now controls the third largest population in the world, one that is addicted to whatever he puts in front of them. There is a tremendous amount of responsibility that comes with that authority. I hope he will respect that responsibility and keep it top of mind when business decisions have to be made.

Days 19–21: Time Off
December 9–10, 2010

Day 22: Red Flags
December 11, 2010
12:35 p.m.

It was one year ago today, nearly to the minute that I walked out of the courtroom with a signed document that allowed me another chance to attempt to live the life I had always dreamed of.

The feeling of a failed marriage is something I can't take lightly. It is the same pain in my heart that comes with the loss of a loved one. The divorce was the death of my dream for a future of a family of my own. The reality that my marriage was better off left as something to grieve rather than to continue on with was the hardest decision of my life.

When I think of December 11, 2010, the day my marriage officially ended, I will always have a flashback to a cool October afternoon sitting approximately five miles off the Lake Michigan shore on my twenty-eight-foot cabin cruiser. It will be a day that will always make me question the decisions I made and the presence of G-d within my life and within this world.

On that October day I was struggling with events that had just recently been revealed to me. I knew I was going to have to confront challenges in my upcoming marriage that had plagued my previous relationships. They were challenges that I knew were beyond my control and beyond my ability to resolve alone. My past experiences had taught me a tremendous amount about the trials and tribulations that I was to encounter moving forward.

It was less than two months until the big day, and I was scared. I did not want to start a new beginning with someone I loved burdened with challenges that I feared we might not be able to overcome. I was heartbroken and afraid, to say the least.

I asked my close friend Bryan, whom I had worked with for the past several years on a daily basis, to take the day off. I needed his guidance. I needed a friend. I trusted Bryan with my life. I trusted his opinion and his perspectives. He trusted me as well. Our lives were so entangled that whatever I was to endure, he would consequentially have to endure it as well.

I used to joke and call Bryan my baseline. I called him that because he knows that I can be a dreamer at times. At other times I allowed my sensitivity to the negativity in the world to bring me down.

If I were excited and acting in a whimsical manner, Bryan would bring my feet back to ground level. If I was beat up and feeling depressed, he would pick me up by giving me a perspective that got me back on my feet. That is why I called him my baseline.

Although I sometimes would push him to dream a little bigger or encourage him to allow me to stay in the clouds for a little longer, his friendship was a gift that I could never thank him enough for. On this October day I needed my friend.

Bryan had taken the afternoon off so we could talk about some of the challenges that were on my plate. We headed over to B Dock at Diversey Harbor, where my boat was sitting for another couple of weeks before all boats had to be out of the water for the season.

I started the boat and we left the harbor. I headed due east toward the middle of nothingness. With the city in the backdrop I kept going until I felt that all of the noise of the city was far in the distance.

I turned off the engine and allowed the boat to just rock. He looked at me and said, "So, you going to tell me what's going on?" I started disclosing to him some of the issues that I had just became aware of that were going to potentially plague my marriage, which was just around the corner. We were both at a loss for words. I was beyond conflicted. We laughed at how in life we never know what is going to get thrown at us. I cried because my heart was shattered. I knew I did not want to start a new beginning with any more obstacles then necessary.

Knowing many of my past experiences and understanding the circumstances, Bryan felt my pain. He definitely understood the dilemma I was in. He had already RSVP'd and he was going to be a member of the wedding party. I told him that I just wanted to put things on hold and try to figure them out, but it was not that easy at this point. We continued to sit, looking at the horizon as the boat rocked.

Bryan looked at me with compassion, feeling my pain and handed me a bottle of Jack Daniels that was sitting in the fridge of the boat's cabin.

"So Ry, what are you going to do?" he asked.

"I don't know," I replied. "I just don't know. I don't want

to get married like this." We each took a short swig of the Jack as we started to stand up and lean on the port side of the boat facing the eastern horizon.

I looked at Bryan with watery eyes and said to him, "Brian, I have no clue which way to go. I don't know if I should just move forward like nothing has changed or if I should call it all off. I know this sounds crazy, but I wish G-d would throw me a sign." Bryan handed me the bottle of Jack and said, "Well, Ry, that's not going to happen; this is in your hands and you're going to have to figure this one out on your own."

Bryan put his arm around my shoulder as his way of telling me that he understood my dilemma and that I was not alone.

We stood quietly gazing out at the horizon for about thirty seconds, and then Bryan pointed down toward the water at a spot near the boat, asking, in a calm tone, "What is that?" There was something that appeared to have an orange glowing reflection about twelve feet below the surface.

"I don't know," I responded.

"Is it a fish? He asked. It started floating closer to the top and was now about seven feet below the surface.

"No," I replied. "It looks like a bag, like an orange plastic grocery bag." We continued staring over the side as this random object was slowly floating upward, moving back and forth with the undertow.

The object reached the surface and sat kissing the port side of the boat. Bryan looked up at me in a state of shock; we were both in disbelief. "It's a red flag. It is literally a big bright red flag!" he called out. Chills went down my spine, and not knowing how to react we both moved quickly into the center of the boat as if we had seen a boogeyman.

Bryan looked at me dead in the eyes and said with an awkward chuckle, "If that is not a sign, then I don't know what is." We were in awe and weirded out, to say the least. Here we were, over five miles from the Chicago shoreline, and a huge red flag had floated up from the water and sat kissing my boat just a couple minutes after my crying out for a sign from the man upstairs.

We left the boat that day overwhelmed by the challenges that I would have to confront. We never talked about that incident to anyone, and I put it in the back of my mind. To me it was just a reminder of the important decisions ahead that were going to have a great affect on my life.

Later that evening I sat down with my fiancée's family. I did what I would want a man marrying my daughter to do—which was to confront their fears.

I did not know which way to move, but I did know that I was in a position that I had never wanted to be in. My wife to be begged, cried, and pleaded with me that she needed me, that we were meant to be together and had promised to do everything as a team to get through this. I gave in to trust and had faith that these challenges were meant to be mine.

I had always felt in my heart that our paths were meant to cross. From the moment I met her everything just felt like we were supposed to be there for each other.

The night that we met, we were at the same bar in Chicago, Rockit Bar and Grill on Hubbard Street. I was there for my cousin's birthday and she was in the same area with a few of her friends. She was only twenty at the time but she still somehow had gotten in the bar.

My best friend and roommate at the time pointed across the bar to her and said, "There you go, Ryan—your wife." With a smile on my face I asked him to repeat himself, and he replied, "Don't act like you don't hear me, go talk to your wife!" I looked at him and said, "After that statement, I guess I have to." I approached the petite little blonde with an innocent bubbly aura radiating from her.

I introduced myself and quickly discovered she was a giggler. It felt so refreshing. I noticed she was with her friends and I said to her after a couple minutes, "Look, you seem like you're having a good time with your friends. Would you be open to giving me your number, and I can call you this week?"

She accepted and I was so excited. I met this sweet and innocent young woman and I was eager to get to know her better. We talked on the phone for a couple of weeks before we hung out. She came over for our first date and I made a nice dinner, working hard to impress her. It was a lemon chicken with artichoke hearts and a pinch of capers, coupled with glasses of white wine.

We watched a movie and just chilled together on the

couch. I was intentionally being passive. I wanted to get to know her, because in the past I had jumped too quickly into situations that I later regretted.

I remember looking over my shoulder at the clock to see what time it was, and she must have thought I was going in for the kiss, because she eagerly reciprocated the gesture. It was an eight-pound kiss. It felt like her whole skull was resting on my lips. Needless to say, it was not the ideal first kiss for either of us. We later would laugh about it often. I guess if I could have judged our relationship from that first kiss, it resembled the heaviness that it was going to later endure.

She called me the next day. I was working in my office, smiling as we talked. She loved to giggle, and it was contagious. I sat staring at this 1950s velvet Einstein painting that had been my grandparent's and had been given to me after my grandmother passed away.

I had a smile on my face talking to this woman who just gave me so much curiosity about the future. She said to me on the phone, "I have a question for you." My first thought was, Uh oh, maybe I once had a bad date with one of her friends; this is going to be over before it even gets started.

"Sure, go ahead," I replied with a nervous confidence.

"Do you know Harriet Beale?" Now, I was really confused.

"Yeah, why? She was my grandmother." She replied that

she had told her mom that she was going out with a Beale from Detroit, and then the gossip chain started: her mom told her grandma about me, and her grandma then told her that she had once had a neighbor named Harriet Beale whom she had been close to. She explained how her grandmother used to walk my father in a stroller sixty-two years earlier.

Here, so many years later, this family was connected to my core. I found out that her great-grandparents and my great-grandparents were friends and had homes next door to each other some eighty years ago.

Every close moment with my grandmother flashed before my eyes. I remembered holding her hand every day when she was unconscious at the hospital, fighting for her life, skipping work just to be there for her, and now in this moment I felt like she was hearing my prayers and sending me signs. I had tears coming down my face. At that moment, I felt that this young woman and I were meant to be. I felt a sense of faith that whatever challenges we were meant to share, they were meant for our growth and this relationship was meant to be.

Before we had met I was going through a phase in which I was feeling somewhat isolated and lonely. I was lacking in my soul a genuine foundation, a closeness of family, a feeling of being loved.

I was single at the time and very good at it. Chicago is a pretty fun place to be for a young single guy. But my friends were all starting to settle down, and I was away from home and getting tired of being alone. I remember a few nights before I met my soon-to-be ex, I was making a prayer. I asked that my grandmother Harriet, who had recently passed away, look out for me and guide me to help me find my *besheret*, which means "meant-to-be"—in other words, my match.

My grandma and I had a very warm and openhearted relationship. I knew that if she could, she would be looking out for me. She was always in my subconscious.

After our first date with this young woman, I was flying high. She was so cute, she had family that lived in the north suburbs of Chicago, and I felt in my heart that she needed me, that I was meant to take care of her.

We dated for almost three years before getting engaged. I was so proud that we were doing it the old-fashioned way. She lived with her parents, and we were waiting until the day of the wedding to start living together. It seemed to me to be ideal.

But soon the visions of a future, a perfect marriage, and a life of fulfillment had faded. Our marriage was full of challenges that we were unable to overcome as a couple.

It was destroying me. I had an ulcer, I was nearly forty pounds overweight, and I had no will to keep fighting. I had lost myself; I had no one to take care of me and I was becoming sick. When the reality of our circumstances had become too much to tuck under the rug, there was a three-month period during which I was unable to look in the mirror without crying. I had such a toxic level of stress that at night I did not think I was going to wake up in the morning. I felt like I was failing G-d's challenge for me. I was lost.

I was so ashamed that I was losing everything that mattered to me. I was so sad about how far I had gone to fight for us and yet I had lost myself in the process. I will never forget looking in that mirror, tears in my eyes, facing constant health problems that I had never had before, and pleading with myself to wake up. I was so far from where I wanted to be that I did not want to live if this was the life I was going to have.

It was one powerful thought that woke me out of what then felt like a life sentence: I said to myself that it is a sin to be sad and it's an obligation to be happy. I was living in sin.

Even though I knew in my heart I was doing everything in my power to save our marriage and that I had done it with the purest intentions, I was still living in sin. As much as I had felt that my marriage was meant to be, I knew that the man upstairs would never condone me living a life as sad and as challenging as mine had become.

I made a pact at that moment, gazing at what was the worst of myself. I promised not to continue to live in sin, being so miserable and losing myself. I was going to take care of my body, my mind, and my heart. I knew that I had to fight for my happiness and I was ready—and deserved—to be happy.

I held on for two more months, though I started working out to get my peace of mind back. I started to see things more clearly every day and I was ready to start living again. The lack of fulfilling love ate away at me, but I still was praying for a miracle, something that would allow me to see the light at the end of the tunnel. No lights came on; just more emptiness. The decisions that I knew I had to make I did not take lightly and I would not make them with a rash state of mind. I made sure that I fought with every ounce of my being to work to resolve the challenges that were plaguing us.

I had met with every person that I could possibly gain insight from to seek out advice I could take back into the home. I had allowed everything in my life that meant something to me to take a back seat to the challenge of trying to save our marriage.

In my heart I knew people would gossip and I would take the rap for unfair criticism, but I was built for it. If enduring unfair criticism because I was an outsider to my wife's community was what needed to be done to clear a better future for her, than that was a sacrifice I was willing to make.

I had to embark on the process of disentangling our marriage. I knew that I was never going to be settled in my heart with the challenges we had endured. We needed to grow up, and unfortunately that meant apart. I felt that this decision was the best chance that we had for the futures that we both wanted for ourselves. Through all of the pain and hardship, I still wanted her to be happy. I knew she would find someone that she could start fresh with and hopefully live the life that she had envisioned for herself.

Once the paperwork was filed, I was naive to think that we could just start healing and moving on with our lives.

The divorce process lasted seven very painful months. I think people were surprised to find out that we did not have anything of value to hold on to or to fight about anymore.

It was seven months that took me away from my own inner peace and from helping to save my brother. It ended today, one year ago, and my life was then given a second chance.

Bryan and I were walking down the street from Wrigley field the other day, and as we were talking we were reliving the devastating tragedies that had taken place. The culmination of events in such a short time frame was beyond our comprehension. For the first time since that cool October afternoon he looked at me, this time with disbelief in his eyes, and in his baseline voice that I have always come to trust he said, "Ry, all I have been thinking about is that red flag."

Days 23–25:
Anticipating the Anniversary
December 12–14, 2010

Day 26: Bittersweet

December 15, 2010

10:04 p.m.

When I first started writing this book and started this project, I was anticipating today. Today was my wedding anniversary. Three years ago today I stood in front of my closest friends and family and took vows for the beginning of a new life. I thought I would be filled with insight and thoughts. The truth is that it genuinely has become an old chapter, and I'm thankful for that at this point in my life. I have more important things to achieve and handle right now.

Yesterday was the Hebrew anniversary of my brother's passing. My parents called this morning to see how I was doing. I felt fine, actually. They went to services and said prayers, and all of us family members lit remembrance candles in our separate homes. What challenges me now is the state of mind my family is in. I am concerned for my father as I think the anniversary has hit him hard. I see him teetering in both his business and his emotions. He has always had the most compassionate, optimistic, and warm outlook on life; that has always radiated to others and inspired people throughout their lives. It was a gift he had. He has always lived for other people, and I see in his eyes that he is challenging himself and questioning if he was a failure. His love and compassion has been shaken. He is questioning his past abilities to be an aggressive businessman and a father figure in these hard economic times, especially hard as they are for the Detroit area. All of these issues come to the top of his mind during this anniversary. Things are good when they are good, but when good cycles break, they break hard. That reality is making my father question himself and his success in his life.

"If it ain't broke, don't try to fix it." But if things are broken and we choose to look the other way, tragic circumstances can creep in and destroy them. I heard today that my dad was walking around his office looking lost. It is the same office that my father, my two brothers, and I all shared once upon a time. It breaks my heart to hear that he is questioning himself and feeling like a failure. Every part of my being wants to make his stress and struggles go away.

If anyone deserves to live a peaceful life and retire, it is my father. He worked selling soda at the state fair grounds when he was in grade school. He never asked for a nickel from his parents. He worked and built businesses. He has always given to charity and has helped support anyone in need, even to a fault. He got into commercial real estate in the early 1970s and started amassing small- and medium-size strip malls. He loved it. He loved helping people get into business so they could provide a living for their families. Every person he came across and worked with was a friend to him. He always treated his employees as if they were business partners.

He never went behind anyone's back and his word was always gold. My father lived this legacy every day and I fear that he is ashamed due to circumstances that grew out of his control. This shame that I fear he is carrying is toxic. It eats away at a person's mind, soul, heart, and pride. He does not deserve this and I am trying to figure out how to help. He needs a spark to launch him into the next chapter of his life. As a son, I feel that—because I do not have my own family today and I can potentially do my business from anywhere—I need to step in. I need to help give him the spark that he has always had. I believe I have what it takes. My challenge is to focus on my dreams and passions while trying to help secure my father's legacy…at least in his heart.

Day 27: Stevie B
December 16, 2010
6:18 p.m.

The past year has been one of the best years and hardest years of my life at the same time. It was the most difficult year of my life because it was filled with tremendous grief and loss. It also pushed me to run so far away from it that I tried to live in the moment as much as possible. When tragedy happens to a loved one, it tends to be a wakeup call that life is fragile and it is not to be taken for granted.

The hardest part within the last year has been accepting the fact that I had seen my brother looking to find calm in his life and I knew that he needed help in which he was too proud to acknowledge. Steve was the brightest star in any room. I know it's nice to say good things about family members, but it was the absolute truth. Nobody could deny that he took over any room he was in. If Steve was at the bar, the owners wanted to take care of him because he brought the people and the energy that they needed for success. If it was a business meeting, when Steve spoke, everyone listened or else they might miss out on the next big opportunity. He radiated confidence and a determination to make things happen. People were mesmerized at his ability to think outside the box and make something out of nothing.

When Steve went to Vegas he would bring all of his close friends and all of the girls that encircled him with love. He would take care of everybody. It was expected. If you thought you were going to try and pay for something, you knew that a war of words would be sure to break out. No matter where he went or where he was, people gravitated toward him. Steve was an ambassador of cultures throughout the Detroit Area and beyond. He brought together Blacks, Whites, Jews, Chaldeans and Arabs. He stood up against injustice and would do everything he could to help those in need. Steve was such a functioning addict with such positive traits and so much potential that his life could have been a case study. Steve always enjoyed having me close by, but he never wanted me to be spoiled by his over extensive generosity. I'm not absolutely sure why, but I believe that he was always trying to teach me a lesson and at times I believe I brought out a sense of insecurity in him.

Steve never wanted anyone to see his inner pain. Being the little brother, this always put me in a tough spot. I have always called things as I've seen them. When I see someone hurting, especially a family member, I have a very hard time turning a cheek. Steve and I often bumped heads because I would not let his big personality overshadow his principals. I often challenged him in ways he had not experienced. Everyone who knew Steve would try to give him some words of advice, but nobody had the courage to truly challenge him. I always challenged him and he always challenged me. He pushed me to be tough and I pushed back to prove a point. He made me want to work harder and be more successful so I could prove to him that I was strong and worthy.

When I saw that over time his big personality had become a shelter for his growing insecure ego, I became worried for what he may do to feed his insecurities. There was no way that he could maintain the momentum that he was building for himself, especially with the challenge of confronting his addictions. His pride was preventing him from dealing with his inner demons. As his friends were settling down and starting families of their own, Steve was finding it harder to find people that would run around town with him looking for stimulation. He was getting lonely; feeling isolated and did not want to accept that the lifestyle he was living was out of balance.

The lessons that I had learned in my failed marriage had taught me a tremendous amount about dealing with our own childhood pain. It taught me about the dangers of tucking grief, anxiety and shame under the rug. Most of us take our hardships and figure a way to put them into a conceptual box so we can accept them quickly in order to move on. Eventually if we just keep moving on without facing our un-dealt with emotions from our past and early childhood, we have a tendency to become unaware of why we react to life events and other people the way that we do.

We hear about it all the time growing up. We hear about how a child who was abused is (x) times more likely to abuse their children. We hear how if your parent or grandparent was an alcoholic than you are (x) times more likely to become an alcoholic. Obviously some of these behaviors are possibly genetic, but there are many behaviors that are learned. Coping mechanisms are also learned and sometimes they are very unhealthy. If a teenager sees that every time their mother gets stressed out she pops an anti-anxiety pill and has a glass of wine, then it would not be uncommon to expect that child to do the same when they have stress.

I had worried about my brother for years. He at times was very aggressive towards people that he loved when he was confronted with stress. Being that I was the youngest of three boys, I witnessed a lot. I also learned a lot, both good and bad behaviors and skills. Steve was seven years older than me, so naturally growing up I always looked to him for encouragement, acceptance and protection at times. As I became older I often worried about him. I worried that his addictive personality was taking its toll on his mind and his body. Over the past few years I had seen him get more fidgety. He always needed several people to be around him. He was afraid to be alone or to even sit alone with someone that may confront his behaviors that were starting to look more out of control.

I remember what had scared me the most. It was his Facebook use. I saw him constantly posting pictures of him doing more and more ridiculous things. I saw it in his eyes. It looked like his soul was lost; always a big bright smile with the same empty eyes. I always had a hard time looking at those pictures. Those were the pictures that started raising the alarms that he needed help. People tend to use Facebook as a way to convince themselves and the people that they are connected with that everything is O.K., even when their world is falling apart. If you look at people's pages, you can often tell who is suffering the most. You can tell by their posts, the type of post that they make, how hard they are trying to smile in their pictures and how often they are posting. I watched my brother slowly decay in his public profile. I am not sure if his friends saw or felt what I saw. The pictures that were being posted were supposed to distract people from seeing what lay under the surface. It's difficult to show honesty about your inner feelings with such a large audience of friends and skeptics; especially if you have an image you are trying to maintain.

Steve suffered because his ego and pride were too large to address and confront his unhealed pain. It was the culmination of years of unhealthy coping behaviors that had built up to a point where he no longer could see the light and the end of the tunnel. In a moment of weakness he took his gun to his right temple and ended his life. I felt like everything I had feared had come true. I watched my brother fight off every time he had an opportunity to challenge his addictive nature. He ducked and dodged all the bullets that came his way since he was seventeen years old and now at thirty seven years of age, he made his final act of control by putting a bullet where his pain and suffering had been nesting, in his head.

For over a year before Steve took his life, the alarm bells had been going off. I had seen the warning signs building up. He had always tried to make it appear that he was drinking less and that he had not been gambling, but I saw that these were all just acts to pacify the critics. I remember a couple years ago he had come into town and the two of us were eating at the Cheesecake Factory off of Michigan Avenue. I watched as his hand was shaking, he was very jittery. Being the little brother that was not afraid to challenge him, I had asked if he was still gambling. I got the same response that you can expect out of someone that is trying to hide something. I got yelled at for even thinking such absurd thought. It did not stop me from still asking for an answer. His answer was "NO! I'm not gambling!".

As we got up to pay the bill, Steve reached into his pocket to grab his cash and out fell his latest betting sheet, with over a dozen weekend games being waged on. He looked at me like a kid who just got caught with his hand in the cookie jar. I just looked back at him with a sense of disappointment. The trust was shaky. I think drinking and whatever recreational things he was doing on the side were taking a toll on his body and his mind. His jitters reminded me of a 75-year-old alcoholic whose liver went to sleep years ago.

Growing up in the same home as my brother I remember when things changed. I remember when Steve changed and our family members took on the roles that a dysfunctional family will take on in order to deal with a tremendous amount of stress to the family system. I had always tried to understand it, but it wasn't until my ex-wife and I had to go through our own lessons that I realized that this was not just about feelings and reactions. There was a science to it and there are tragic results for families and individuals who do not properly confront their vicious cycles. Knowledge is power and the knowledge that I had learned had taught me what I was always feeling, but did not understand. My family was dealing with unresolved grief and Steve found ways to avoid dealing with pain that nested for years.

Through my marriage I had learned that a family in dysfunction would take on four roles to cope. These roles are the Hero, the Scapegoat, the Mascot and the Lost Child. As I understand it, all four roles will be taken on no matter how many family members there are. At times, family members may shift roles inadvertently. I once heard the analogy that the family system is like a wind chime. On an average day it sits calm and makes a little music. Some days the winds pick up and when the system is in harmony they will make music together. Once in a while a big storm will come through and knock the wind chime around and it will become entangled and unable to function properly without spending the energy to disentangle it. In life, tragedies can and will strike and can knock us out of harmony as well.

I believe looking back this is what happened in our family. I can only speak to my generation, but I believe that it goes back generations. I'll never forget that one night when I was seven years old and laying in my parents' bed. The phone rang and my mom answered. Her hands rose to her face as the phone dropped and the loudest scream that I had ever heard came charging out of her. It was that moment that my family's wind chime got entangled. The call was from my aunt, she said that my mom's brother was found dead, hanging. He was 38 years old. Almost the same exact age that Steve was when he died. Our family was never 100 percent settled on the events that had taken place that had led up to my uncle's death. Some felt it was accidental, some felt that there was foul play involved. The bottom line was, we lost an uncle, my mom lost a brother and our family was broken.

Steve was fourteen at the time. He and my uncle were very close. They use to go for Sunday rides on my uncle's motorcycle and my uncle was the one who kept our family in harmony. My uncle would throw regular barbecues and always added a sense of fun and silliness to the occasion, much like how my brother had. I could never recall a time prior that there was not harmony in the home before my uncle had passed. After my uncle had passed, things changed. I think this is when we went into these roles that I only recently had learned about. I wish we could have understood these roles earlier so we could have been more aware of how we were dealing with our grief.

Steve took on the Hero role. He was the big brother and wanted to be tough. He wanted to be a rock to me and my other brother. But he never expressed how he was feeling besides displaying acts of anger. Steve started getting into fights in school and when he would get mad he would tear up the house. His inner feelings of rage would come out through a dominating personality that he started to take on.

My other brother, I believe took on the role of the Mascot. The Mascot has lots of friends, spends little time at home and tends to go with the flow. The Mascot also tends to avoid angry confrontations and learns ways to entertain the family so they can be distracted from dealing with the grief. My middle brother got into magic. He loved it. He became so involved in magic that he would never miss any of the big performers that came into town and he knew hundreds of tricks. I was always proud to be the magician's assistant. When I learned about these roles, I had my *Aha!* Moment. It was us. It is hard to be objective. However, I believe I took on the role of the scapegoat with a little bit of the Lost Child. The scapegoat is often times argumentative, seeks attention and senses the heaviness of the guilt within the family. The Lost Child tends to become a loner, withdraws from others and is uncomfortable with any kind of real attention. I think I was somewhere in the middle of the two. I definitely had depression that I was dealing with as my family had been shaken at its core.

As time went on Steve was introduced to gambling and that became an outlet. It became an activity that created a significant amount of arousal and stimulation. All three of us were enchanted by the game and we had friends that enjoyed the gambling bug as well. Some of the friends had more control than others, but Steve never knew his limits or he always pushed beyond the safe zone. My parents did their best to address the issues as they came up, but they were never fully aware of where they had evolved. Within a few years of my uncle's passing, my father was diagnosed with non-invasive bladder cancer and my mother had been diagnosed with an Acoustic Neuroma, a benign brain tumor. These new life-threatening challenges overshadowed everything else. Thank G-d my mom had the tumor removed and my father was able to beat the cancer, but by this time the suppressed emotions of the past were lost in history.

This is where I think every person has a vulnerability to getting lost or forgetting where the root of his or her emotional wounds lay. Life goes on and new challenges arise; yet true closure from the past is long forgotten. Who wants to talk about the past, right? Well, I believe the past holds the keys to true healing and understanding. I always thought that Steve was holding on to that anger and rage of losing our uncle and I never knew how to approach that conversation. I remember not too long after learning about how family members can take on these roles that I was at dinner with my brother and his girlfriend at the time. I was explaining to her about the family system and how life events can play a significant role into our personalities and how we tend to take on roles to cope with our grief. I was sharing with her about our own family experience and how I believed that when my uncle was found dead, it affected us. Before I could finish my sentence Steve raised his voice and roared, "HE WAS MURDERED!!". That was the first time in my entire life that I had ever heard him say anything about it. At that moment I knew that his rage was deep and unsettled.

When I buried my brother, his plot laid right next to my uncle's. My uncle a Vietnam veteran, dead at 38 years of age, my brother dead at thirty-seven and a half; that was no coincidence in my mind.

Days 28-30: Left to Grow
December 17-19, 2010

Day 31: Reunions

December 20, 2010

5:27 p.m.

I'm packing up to go to Michigan tomorrow morning for Christmas break. It has been a little harder to write because thankfully I have had more peace of mind lately. It usually takes a good amount of anxiety to get the most out of putting pen to paper. Today was a mix of several emotions. It was last year that I was packing to go to Michigan, eager to see my brothers, nephews, and sister-in-law, as well as my parents. I was packing the same suitcase when I got the call that my brother had taken his life. A lot has changed in the last year.

Tomorrow I will see my nephews and the rest of my family. I guess it is the same, minus the funeral and mourning, but we will still be minus one. I was just packing and came across my wedding video. I was debating for a while over the last year to get rid of it but I could not. I kept it because it has five minutes of my brother giving me the greatest speech as my best man. I just watched it. When he first came on my heart sunk, but then the pain subsided. I watched him looking like "the man." He was saying kind words and giving me credit for my accomplishments—words I had dreamed my whole life he would say to me one day. I always wanted to impress my big brother. He was my toughest critic. Watching the video made me realize that even through all of the hardship of a failed union I would have paid every penny I had for those few moments; at least I got those.

Going home tomorrow leaves me with several questions of how it is going to be. How is my family going to feel as we relive the anniversary of my brother's death? How are people going to respond or even react knowing that it has been one year? People knew my brother and they loved him. He was one of the most popular people in southeast Michigan, and even that could be an understatement. I am looking forward to seeing my family. I am also looking forward to seeing an amazing and strong young woman I've met. I'm cautiously optimistic. I have had to maintain the balance between allowing myself to fall in love and allowing myself to keep my feet on the ground. All signs indicate that this could be someone to share my life with. Over the past month we have talked on the phone for over two hours a night. My motivation to meet other women has subsided and I still hold myself from fully falling.

I am a romantic by nature. I know from past experience that I have allowed red flags to just pass by unnoticed, so I am trying to restrain myself. It kind of sucks having to hold back, because the best part of falling in love is the fall. This time around I want to have someone that I *like* more than I love. The love is like a drug, with highs and lows. I know that if I like sharing myself with someone who respects me, treats me well, and likes me as much as I like being with her then I can fall in love slowly for the rest of my life. It is more important to have a best friend and partner rather than just someone you love. I have loved several people that were toxic for me and if I do not learn from my mistakes, I will be deserving of the headaches that come from learning all over again. That is my balance right now. I need to let go enough to allow myself to love but, more important, to allow myself to be loved.

Days 32–35:

Spending time with the family and getting to know my new lady friend

December 21–24, 2010

Day 36: Living Moments
December 25, 2010
4:10 p.m.

It was one year ago yesterday that I was packing my bag, excited to go to Michigan to see my family over Christmas break. My brother and sister in-law from North Carolina were coming into town with my nephews, and we were all going to be together. It has been an extremely hard year for me. Every day I felt like I was battling to keep my sanity. My marriage had been a disaster, full of the fear of waiting for the next curve ball to come out of left field and hit me in the face. Amazingly, the divorce was even more dramatic. I had people pulling strings and playing legal games, motivated only by revenge, anger, and financial gain.

At the time it had been surreal that I finally was in control of my own life following the finalized divorce. A sense of a new beginning had begun to take over my spirit and I was so looking forward to the following day and sharing this new me and new life with all of my family. I was packing, feeling a sense of freedom and renewal that I had not felt in years, when I got the call. My oldest brother had taken his life. I could not tell if this was a bad dream I was having or if I was awake. I called my mom and asked her, "Is this a dream or is this real?"

"Yes, Ryan, it's real," she replied.

"OK," I said in a subtle, calm voice. I hung up the phone and in a trancelike state continued packing.

I remember telling myself, *Now I need a suit*, and I

calmly packed one. I needed a tie, so I walked into my closet and grabbed a tie. I stood still in the moment and was not sure if this was a dream or real life. I started calling my close friends one by one to see if I could get pinched to wake up. No one answered the phone. It was nearly an hour before someone called me back. That was one of the hardest hours of my life. I was alone, not sure if this was real. Then my phone started ringing, people had seen messages all over Facebook about my brother's death. E-mails were blasted, people were posting on my wall, and it was out of control.

If I had not answered the phone call from my brother Sam calling to tell me about Steve's passing, I would have heard the news via a Facebook wall post. The thought of that still makes me shiver. Things were put into high gear at that moment and my body was taken over by anxiety, anger, rage, and denial. I remembered the Haganah head instructor and founder, the message he always posted: "SUB –Soldier Up, B**ch!" Straight to the point. Just as I was starting to catch my breath from having the life snatched out of me, real life was about to start.

It was going to start with another test. I knew I had to be aware that I needed to keep my sanity, help my family, and not lose faith for a better tomorrow. It was not easy, but when a challenge or a decision had to be made I took the path of tackling it head on. When the funeral home asked if anyone wanted to speak on my brother's behalf, I volunteered. I delivered a eulogy that I wrote in twenty minutes that summed up the life, the passion, and the struggles my brother lived and died with.

Two nights ago there was a lecture in my brother's honor.

The topic was "How to Remain Calm When Everyone around You Is Going Crazy." It was about being codependent, but also being a strong individual and more or less knowing oneself. A couple hundred people showed up, including my friend's mom, the friend whose brother had just died. A rabbi and author gave the lecture, which was amazing. It hit upon everything that my family had been discussing earlier that day. My family sat in the front row and chuckled at how relevant the lecture was to the crisis we were living with, a crisis that we will live with and deal with for the rest of our lives. At the end I felt uplifted and empowered. I knew that several people in the room that night were going to take something with them, at least a seed of understanding that could empower the rest of their lives.

After the lecture, they were selling the Rabbi's books, and he was also signing them. I picked one up and, not caring too much about getting his autograph, went to thank him for delivering such a great message. I told him that I wanted to thank him, that he had given the perfect speech, with perfect timing and the perfect delivery. He said he was honored to have received such a rewarding response. He asked my name, as well as if I would like him to sign the book. I said sure. I told him my name and he paused. He said, "Did you write a speech and eulogy for your brother Steve?" I told him that I had. He said that someone had forwarded the speech to him and that it was the premise and inspiration for the message he gave in his lecture. I was moved to see how our positive actions in times of struggle come full circle. I was empowered by the message he delivered at just the right time in my life, a message that was in turn inspired by a moment of courage I had had a year earlier.

Although memories of the past have the power to influence our todays and tomorrows, we have a choice in every moment to plant a seed that can inspire us for the future.

Days 37–38: Enjoying Life
December 26–27, 2010

Day 39

December 28, 2010

10:37 a.m.

I realized yesterday, after checking my calendar, that tomorrow will be my fortieth day. I tried to ask myself what this means. I have not looked back at what I have written and I have questioned if there will be any relevance to anyone who may read this.

I always wanted to write with the intention of putting something out to the world that could plant a seed for a more positive future. I mean, that is what has always driven me to writing, that potential and power. That's why they say that the pen is mightier than the sword.

I hope and pray that my tribulations will open others minds to reflect on their experiences with new eyes. The past few weeks have been full of new life, new meaning, and hope for a brighter tomorrow. I look at where I am today, still drinking a coffee and waiting for my breakfast to come. My perception has calmed. I feel that the purpose of starting this personal journey has been fulfilled. I feel at ease; I have no doubt embarked on my life's next chapter. Still, small dramas from the past linger; but the power of a new beginning is much stronger as a force pushing forward than the past is at pulling me back.

I have begun to fall for a woman who I feel can make me a better man. I have found direction and strategy for work, and I have begun reconciling with old friends.

Day 40
December 29, 2010

4:05 p.m.

When I started this project I was at a point of surrender. My life and reality had turned upside down in what seemed like overnight. I had lost my marriage, I had lost my dream office, I had to walk away from my comfortable three-story Chicago walk-up, I had fallen into debt for the first time since college. I had lost my brother, and I was looking for a home for my puppy because I could no longer provide the sort of home that a growing Old English Sheepdog deserved.

Life had reminded me that nothing is permanent, but with faith, discipline, and determination I could keep fighting knowing that one day this could all become a memory of a chapter of resilience.

I had to wrestle with my mind not to give in to fear and not to give up. I had to be an ark and rise above the flooding waters, for one day they would subside and the lessons learned would permeate my being.

When life happens, whether it is the death of a loved one, losing a home, or even winning the lottery, we have choices to make. Are we going to be aware enough not to get drowned, or are we going to be an ark? If we choose to be an ark, we can stay above the waters so we can assess the damage and where we want to land when the flood subsides. Life is always better than no life, no matter the circumstances and even though today's challenges may feel like they are drowning us, so long as we have breath we can begin to envision where our ark is going.

When I look back to when I started this journey, I try to see the man that I was and what has changed today. I gauge what I have been able to accomplish since my forty days began.

In the past forty days, I traveled to Florida to spend time with my grandmother and family. I spent time in Charlotte, North Carolina, with my brother, sister-in-law, and beautiful nephews. I traveled to Michigan four times and have helped my father get back on pace with his business and refocus his life goals. I have helped focus and give direction to my businesses, which I have been working to take to the next level. I met an amazing woman who has since become my girlfriend.

Yet, I realize the landscape around me has changed permanently. Today I sit at new crossroads, wondering which direction my life shall go. When I started this journey, I never thought I would be where I am today in such a short period of time.

The last few days I have been wondering how my purpose relates to where I am. I live in Chicago, yet my notion of the quality of life here versus the quality of life that I can attain by living somewhere else, for the first time since living here, has shifted.

I am once again looking forward to the future.

Personal Pivot Events since I Finished My Forty Days

I realize that often times we have an expectation to seek out immediate results from our efforts. However, it is important to appreciate that it is the seeds that we plant in our past that bear the fruit for our future. The following events are what I like to call *Pivotal Events;* for me they were life changing.

These are events that are shaping my future today and have significantly affected my life. These events are not all moments of joy, but they are all filled with a deep and genuine passion that was awakened during my forty days off. I see them as meaningful moments along my journey.

February 22, 2011

Said, "I love" you to my girlfriend cautiously for the first time, my guard is slowly coming down.

March 15, 2011

Packed all of my belongings into a twenty-four-foot U-Haul and moved back home to Michigan. I'd miss Chicago, my home for the past eight and a half years, but my family needed me and I needed them. On the other hand, there was a woman back in Michigan who had begun to capture my heart.

May 2011

Applied to the Pepsi Refresh Project to win $50,000 to work toward mental health awareness in our society, under the title "Rock your Mind with Pure Mental Graffiti." The top ten projects will win the grant.

June 1, 2011

I realized that my girlfriend and I have been living together since I moved back to Michigan. It dawned on me when someone asked if we lived together. My answer had been no, but we soon realized that since I had moved back we had only spent one night apart. We "officially" started living together after that.

June 8, 2011

My girlfriend and I packed the car, threw a tent and a sleeping bag in the trunk, and strapped two beach cruiser bicycles on the car and started driving. It was a true American road trip.

June 11, 2011

We left Charlotte, North Carolina abruptly after I had a bizarre blow-up with my brother Sam and my sister-in-law. Unsettled feelings came to the surface.

June 29, 2011

Received an e-mail from Pepsi. The "Pure Mental

Graffiti" proposal was accepted, and now I would need to spam my Facebook friends to let them know that I was officially competing in July's Pepsi Refresh Project.

July 1, 2011

Craziness began, figuring our strategy to finish in the top ten in the Pepsi Refresh Project and win $50,000 in honor of my brother Steve and those with mental health problems who need to be reached.

Early July 2011

Dumpster diving for yellow Pepsi bottle caps. Raiding the stands at Comerica Park after the game. Whoring out my Facebook friends and begging family and friends to do the same. Spending 100-degree days in Walmart's outdoor bottle return centers and at recycling plants.

July 22, 2011

We were in tenth place and looking strong.

July 24, 2011

The puppy shelters teamed up against us and won five of the top ten spots.

July 31, 2011

We finished in fifteenth place out of three hundred entrants in the $50,000 category of ideas that got accepted for the Pepsi Refresh Project. We brought a lot of great attention toward fighting the stigma behind mental health and increasing awareness. We received tons of calls of support from people all over the country. Local papers wrote about the cause. All in all, we got people talking. It was a win.

August 10, 2011

My girlfriend officially deleted her Facebook page and discovered she was happier and less anxious then she had ever been in her past. I kept mine for business and the ability to be a voyeur for when it was needed.

August 30, 2011

After realizing that the heaviness of the last few years had left my demeanor with a heavy feel, I signed up for a six week, stand-up comedy class. I graduated today by performing for five minutes in front of a crowd of nearly three hundred spectators. It was something I always wanted to do. It was a great outlet and I'm working on getting the lighthearted side of me back. I'm working on my funny.

September 2011

Opened a private gym and started teaching martial arts locally to private classes and small groups. It's always been a healthy part of my life and I was happy to be able to now pursue this passion in Detroit.

December 20, 2011

I proposed to my girlfriend; she said yes!

December 21st 2011

My girlfriend's parents were very excited. The engagement started as something that was filled with love and excitement and then quickly moved on to something filled with anxiety and stressful expectations.

December 26, 2011

Today I had to take on a responsibility I never imagined I would have to confront. My father was dealt an unfavorable business proposition. After he hit a mental wall, I was asked to step in and separate my father from the quiet chaos that was unfolding.

This day and the months that followed were tough. We all felt the grief of this reality, but yet we had to fight to find the light at the end of the tunnel.

When they had closed my brother's casket two years earlier I knew this day was eventually going to come. It almost felt as if this is what Steve was preparing me to be tough for. His tattoo and his headstone read LOVE ALL, TRUST FEW. I had never understood what the hell compelled him to get that tattoo. This day brought me to understand that deeper message. It was a very sad day in my family's history.

March 26, 2012

My fiancée and I decided to fight for our dreams. We hopped on a plain to Israel with the hope to get married.

We left our parents a video DVD explaining where we would be. We decided to jump head first into faith at this point in our life and hoped the man upstairs would catch us.

April 5, 2012

We got married on the roof of King David's garden. We shared our vows on the top of Mount Zion overlooking the city of Jerusalem. Both of our parents showed up, as well as my wife's brother and nearly a hundred other relatives. We had a professional photographer, a videographer, a seven-piece klezmer band, and thousands of observers. We had dozens of rabbis, priests, nuns, and people from dozens upon dozens of nations watch as we married. It was the day before Passover, which is also known as the day of Jesus' Last Supper. The city of Jerusalem was packed, and as my new father-in-law recalls it, it was the most amazing flash wedding in the world. It was nothing short of a miracle. The whole thing was one giant blessing. It by far, was the best day of my life.

June 2012

By this time I was fully engaged in working to help stabilize my father's peace of mind. His lifetime of work got crushed to pieces in the failing of Michigan's economy over the past five years. The people who he had always taken care of were now too hungry for their own needs to remember the lifetime of generosity my father always shared. Without dreams and purpose we are lost and die. My father is trying to remember what it was like to dream. I am trying to lead by example.

August 30, 2012

My wife and I closed on the purchase of our first home.

October 18, 2012

My wife and I met her birth mother for the first time. It was one of the most amazing moments of life coming full circle that I have ever witnessed. When they saw each other their bodies shook; they hugged for a while and tears came. They laugh alike. I knew that my wife always dreamed of what this day might be like or feel like. It was an honor and a gift to help watch her dream come to fruition. She had always felt blessed for being adopted, but there had also always been a small void in her heart. When I asked her that night how she felt, she told me that for the first time the void was no longer there.

November 3, 2012

My wife took a pregnancy test and it came back positive. Life is moving forward.

November 19, 2012

We went to the doctor and saw our little bean, who had a strong heart beat. It is a miracle that I am just starting to try to put my head around. Looking back I cannot believe the gifts that life is giving me. I still feel like it's not real, that a part of me is still sitting in my Chicago apartment trying to figure out where to go from here.

November 22, 2012

Thanksgiving day, three years since the last time I was with my brother Steve. I stayed cuddled in bed with my wife and our little bean, watching movies most of the day. I cried quite a bit and vented my frustration at the fact that my family, after all of our tragedy, was further apart than ever.

My mother was in Florida, prepping my grandmother to move back to Michigan, as she had reached the point at which she could no longer live alone. My brother, sister-n-law, and kids remained in Atlanta and unfortunately we have remained more distant than ever. My father was waiting to hear about what time we were going to my wife's family's house. I have always tried, every day, to say thanks and be thankful. This Thanksgiving I felt very blessed, but my heart was aching for what was missing. I guess the moral of the story is that we must appreciate our blessings every day. It's easy to look outside, scroll on a page and see life in the perfect way that others want us to see it. It is much more challenging to look within, appreciate the good, and do our best to live the life that we were meant to lead.

A life full of dreams, a life full of trying, and a life full of laughing and crying is what we must aspire to. When life is void of ascending toward our dreams we must ask ourselves what we are chasing. Maybe it's worth forty days to try to figure that out.

Ryan G. Beale

How My Life Has Changed Since I Started This Journey

Over the past two years I have done three interventions, in which I can say that people's lives were in the direct line of fire. I have also helped nearly a half a dozen people that I love open their minds to breaking out of the toxic cycles they have been in.

The reality is that we all have our own emotional battles, and usually when we start to confront them we begin to realize at a new level how dysfunctional our own families are or were. And yes, I am confident that every family system can use a little TLC. We should not spend a lifetime trying to figure out why we are all a little crazy, but it is critical to understand why it is that we can, at times, drive other people crazy.

Our challenge is to become more self-aware. When we are in emotional pain, we turn our learned defense mechanisms on in an attempt to control our anxiety. I look at anxiety as a personal power plant. Everything starts with a few ants in the pants. Anxiety makes us want to go outside when the sun is shining; it makes us want to make a better living for ourselves and our family; it makes us *not* want to sit still, but to instead move forward with life.

When times get challenging or life throws us tragedy, anxiety tends to be stronger than we can sustain, and maintaining a healthy balance seems impossible. Life is going to throw us tragedy and give us pain. That is one thing that is guaranteed. I do not mean to put a dark shadow on the journey, but it is within these times of pain that a more meaningful pursuit and journey can be born.

These are the times when we must confront our emotions, reflect upon ourselves, and try not to follow conventional wisdom. If we do not allow these moments of high anxiety and high trauma to breathe properly, we allow the fire of their pain to burn us internally. We naturally crave control, and when life gets a little out of control, in an attempt to regain balance we tend to become controlling, and the worst byproduct of this is the inflicting of our pain on other people.

The reality is that in times like these, there is more at stake than ever. When a genuine loving hug is hard to give and even harder to receive, there is a problem.

When we sense that we have a veil connecting ourselves from the world or we need to take something (pills, alcohol, drugs) to remove that veil, to loosen our inhibition in order to "feel" and "enjoy" the world around us, this is a red flag. This is when we have a choice to make. The ball is in our court and the game is our life. Are we going to sit still until our clock runs out and the buzzer goes off? I say that we must start to dribble the ball slowly, start feeling the ball bounce a little, and slowly make our way toward our goal.

We can choose to accept that everybody is who he or she is. We can believe that nobody changes. We can keep our emotions bottled up, have surface conversations, and attempt to have a genuine relationship in the interests of formality. The other option is to change ourselves by opening up and working to nurture and allow the fire within us to breathe properly and potentially become a place of warmth and light for others.

When we choose to acknowledge the issues and emotional walls that exist, the voids that make us numb at best, or mean, painful, and angry at other times, can be healed. We must choose to work on them so we can have a healthy meaningful relationship with others and ourselves—relationships that can help us grow to a new level of happiness.

The choice to move forward toward our goals sounds wonderful, but it means that we have to dribble past the guards; honest conversations and revelations will occur. Self-reflection and education must be done at an individual level, and we must work with those on our team. We have to learn what it means to be emotionally nurturing to ourselves and others at a healthy and balanced level.

The byproduct of your decision in times of challenge will be growth and love, and a closer, healthier, and happier family. You and your family members and friends will all reap the benefits of this newfound balance. We all need a little luck, a lot of faith, and to know that we *never* walk alone.

Epilogue:
Facebook Officially Goes Public

May 18, 2012
6:10 p.m.

The media airwaves were filled with anticipation in the weeks leading up to today, when Facebook officially became a publicly traded company. With over 900 million active users throughout the world, the value of the initial public offering (IPO) was launched at approximately $86 billion. It is one of the largest IPOs in the history of the stock market, and Facebook's initial value is greater than that all of the S&P 500 companies combined. Now the challenge is how to continue to monetize Facebook's audience. I give Mark Zuckerberg credit for his talents in being able to so precisely execute his ideas. I even bought forty shares when it went public, just to have my hand in history. I sold the shares less than ten minutes later at a loss.

Facebook is, to me, like Pandora's box. The power of the beast has been unleashed. It has allowed us to connect to people that we thought we would never see again. It has empowered political revolutions to occur at lightning speeds. It really is an unbelievable force that has made its mark in history.

The part that affects me in my heart is that there are 900 million people out there who are searching for something that Facebook will never give them. Are we really all supposed to be connecting and sharing everything we do, with everybody we have ever come in contact with? For me, looking back, it has felt so empty. Facebook has connected me to so many people, yet my friendships have not gained any significant value. My family is less close, although most of us are on Facebook. My phone rings less often, and conversations with the ones I care about most have dissipated. It would not be inappropriate to put the burden of these challenges in direct relation to the rise of social networking.

Only time will tell if the world will become more connected and a better place because of Facebook. As I close this up today, the world is at odds. Cultures are on a collision course on a scale like never before. More people are connecting with each other at a faster rate than at anytime in history, yet at the same time we are more divided on our direction as a civilization than ever before.

The world has changed. My hope is one day, when I have kids, they will understand that there was once a time that the family sat and had dinner together with no interruptions. There was once a time that a heartfelt moment was embraced and not just "shared" through social media. More importantly, it is those moments that we may forget about in the future that added the real spiritual value to our sense of being. Some would even go as far to say that it is those precious moments that life is all about.

I know I am unable to change the world alone, but I can start on my own level, tonight in my home. As I close off this journey I am thankful to be able to share a nice peaceful Friday night dinner with my wife. I will end the same way that I started, with a moment of reflection and a prayer. I will pray that G-d will continue to grant me the strength to accept the things that I cannot change, the courage to change the things I can and the wisdom to know the difference. I have faith that nothing in this world is just by chance; and that these words that have come from my experience were intended to be shared with *you*.

A Gift For You

The next forty pages are the most meaningful pages within this book. They are intentionally left blank as my gift to you. These pages are waiting for you to challenge yourself to look within. I have found that keeping a journal is one of the most powerful and rewarding gifts that we, as intellectual beings, can experience.

A journal does not judge. It does not discriminate by age, gender, race, religious affiliation or personal experience. It can be private or it can be celebrated.

Keeping a journal is the first step in bringing your thoughts, ideas and experiences into the material world. It takes something that is invisible and gives it life. It empowers the keeper to evolve by reflecting and sharing if they so choose.

Just think; what distraction in your life, in which by taking forty days away from, will enable you to connect better to your core? Challenge yourself by taking just three minutes to start to look within. You can start off with, "Today I feel…" and the rest is up to you.

I wish you the best in your journey-

Ryan G. Beale

Day 1

Day

Day

Day

Day

Day

Day

Day

Day

Day

Day____

Day

Day

Day

Day

Day

Day

Day

Day

Day

Day

Day

Day

Day

Day _____

Day

Day

Day

Day ___

Day

Day

Day

Day

Day

Day

Day

Day

Day

Day

Day

Day

(ATTENTION)
To Those Who Took The Challenge

If you were one of the lucky individuals who chose to take the forty-day challenge, there may be someone out there whose life can be positively impacted from your efforts. Everybody has a unique journey and a unique story to tell. Often times we tend to open up and learn the most when we see, hear or read how someone else's experience had affected them.

If you are one of the brave souls that would like to share your story or even just a snap shot of your experience please contact us @ 40daysoff.com

40daysoff.com will be accepting stories from individuals who choose to share their experience.

CPSIA information can be obtained
at www.ICGtesting.com
Printed in the USA
FSHW012352050219

9 780989 246040